NATURALLY BEAUTIFUL

First published in the United States of America in 1999
by UNIVERSE PUBLISHING
A Division of Rizzoli International Publications, Inc.
300 Park Avenue South
New York, NY 10010

99 00 01 02/ 10 9 8 7 6 5 4 3 2 1

Printed in England

Designed by Ronni Ascagni, Ascagni Design Inc.

Library of Congress Catalog Card Number: 99-71278

NATURAL BEAUTIFUL

earth's secrets and recipes for skin, body, and spirit

DAWN GALLAGHER

TEXT BY MELANIE MENAGH

UNIVERSE

Foreword by Jill Goodacre Connick

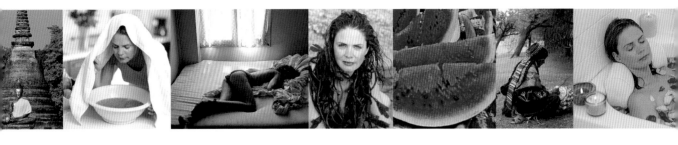

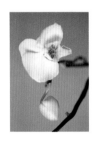

FOREWORD

I have known Dawn Gallagher for fifteen years, and I'm proud to call her my friend. I've always regarded her as someone who places the well being of the environment at the forefront of her agenda. She has discovered the proper balance between utilizing the earth's resources and protecting them.

Herbal hair infusions, avocado masks, and cucumber toners are all examples of Dawn's dedication to achieving beauty in a natural way, while avoiding the use of chemicals that are dangerous not only to us but to our delicate ecosystem. Equally impressive is Dawn's awareness of world beauty. She is blind to creed, code, color, and cult. Beauty is beauty. What a wonderful thing to celebrate and preserve.

The information in this book is the result of years of dedicated research. I am sure the reader will enjoy its insights and surprises, to be followed by a lifetime of natural, healthful living.

JILL GOODACRE CONNICK

Skin as clear as water,
Eyes white as milk,
Back as long, firm
And straight as a
Young Acacia tree

Wodabe tribal song of feminine beauty
Niger, traditional

In every era, in every country and culture, poets have sung of beautiful women as creatures of nature. In this African song, skin is as fine and precious as water. For a Renaissance poet, lilies and roses shone in a fair lady's face. The heroes of the Hindu Vedas saw all the stars of the heavens in their loves' eyes. Although the concept of ideal beauty changes over time and from place to place, beauty has always been equated with the natural world. Every woman is beautiful because she is a part of nature.

The mission of this book is to offer women an array of natural body care ideas that will evoke individual, inner radiance. These chapters cull recipes and techniques from around the world—a facial cleanser from Tahiti, body treatments from Persia, hair conditioners from Mexico, a foot massage from China—so that you can experiment, try whatever intrigues you, and ultimately develop a total body care plan that is custom made by you, for you.

It is only recently, in industrialized societies, that women have depended on preparations sold by multi-national corporations. Traditionally, women devised their own beauty regimens and mixed and produced their own cosmetics. Recipes were passed down in peasant families or villages, tested and refined by each generation; or they might be secret formulas of a shaman or priestess, reserved for religious leaders or royalty on ceremonial occasions.

Whether pharaoh or farmwife, people for tens of thousands of years have used potions derived from natural substances found in the forests, meadows, and oceans around them: grasses, flowers, milk, ores, tree bark, fruit, seaweed, clay. Archeologists have uncovered body-painting pigments made from plants and minerals at Paleolithic sites, leading to speculation that cosmetics came before clothes. These painted adornments, used by both men and women, were probably part of religious rituals and endowed with magical properties.

Equipment for distilling essential oils and containers with traces of perfume dating back five thousand years have been found in Pakistan. Most likely, the Mesopotamians and Chinese were producing aromatic oils by the following millennium. The Egyptians had a vast assortment of products and techniques to enhance beauty and prolong youth: precious bathing and massage oils made from aloe and almond, and kohl made from soot and metallic ores to accentuate the eyes and brows. A twenty-five-hundred-year-old mummy was unearthed in Peru with a complete set of toiletries, including a powder puff made of feathers, to beautify the deceased in the hereafter.

The Greeks, of course, worshiped the body and believed that cold baths improved fitness and vigor; they scrubbed down with goat's fat soap and followed baths with olive oil massages. The Romans collected rich herbs and unguents from all over their far-flung empire and put them to good use at enormous public baths, several of which occupied more than one million square feet. The baths had gardens, restaurants, and theaters, and offered a host of luxurious amenities: hot and cold baths, steam rooms, and massages.

In China, court ladies created porcelain-pale complexions with rice powder. Eyebrows were plucked and redrawn. Elaborate hairstyles were adorned with jade ornaments. Feet were bound and fingernails were elongated with jeweled nail guards. The Chinese system of medicine, based on the opposing principles of yin and yang, used soothing herbal preparations to promote health and beauty.

The *Kama Sutra*, India's guide to lovemaking, enjoins women to learn many methods of pleasing their partners. The text also includes specific recipes for cosmetics, fragrant oils, and henna pastes. These were to be applied liberally to all parts of the body, darkening the teeth, scenting the navel, and coloring the soles of the feet. Buddhism and Ayurveda promoted a balance of body and spirit through exercises, meditation, aromatherapy, diet, and herbal preparations.

In Persia, Islam demanded a strict regimen of ablution, aided by perfumed oils and unguents, as a sign of purity and holiness. Arab physicians tested and wrote extensively about the healing and beautifying power of plants. The celebrated tenth-century scientist Avicenna wrote an entire book on uses for the rose and developed highly effective methods for distilling essential oils.

How can I tell of the rest of creation . . .
Shall I speak of the manifold and various loveliness of sky, and earth, and sea;
of the plentiful supply and wonderful qualities of the light, of sun, moon, and stars;
of the shade of trees, of the colors and perfume of flowers; of the multitude of birds,
all differing in plumage and in song; of the variety of animals,
of which the smallest in size are often the most wonderful—the works of ants
and bees astonishing us more than the huge bodies of whales?

Saint Augustine
Algerian, 4th to 5th century
from *The City of God*

Public and private bathing continued to flourish in the Middle Ages. European alchemists experimented with extracting processes to produce herbal infusions and perfumed oils. Crusaders brought back exotic flowers, scents, and spices from the East—as well as a taste for luxury. A medieval bath often involved a banquet served to men and women sitting in vats of warm water infused with soothing, sweet-scented herbs, and entertainment provided by jesters and musicians. Nearby, bed chambers were at the ready should the proceedings take a more amorous turn.

During the Renaissance, bathing went out of fashion, due to church injunctions against public displays of the body and the fear of disease. People disguised pox and plague spots with face powder, and malodors with scent. A class of professional perfumers sprang up, catering to the nobility and emerging bourgeoisie. Europeans' "discovery" of new lands yielded an entire hemisphere's worth of new and efficacious plants at the disposal of the cosmetic artisans of Paris and Venice.

Self-adornment reached dizzying heights. The less people bathed, the more they covered themselves with powder, paint, and patches. Elaborate makeup, wigs, and clothing rendered the real person barely recognizable beneath the artifice. By the nineteenth century, the romantic movement in Europe and America promoted a return to nature, and Victorian middle-class sensibilities turned away from baroque excesses. At the same time, advances in science and the industrial revolution meant that, for the first time, commercial cosmetics could be made from synthetic materials.

Even though cosmetics was an established trade, it wasn't until after World War II that large-scale chemical manufacturers came to dominate the industry. By the close of the century, things had come full circle, as the major beauty care companies, reacting to consumer demand, began reformulating their products to include natural, nonsynthetic ingredients.

SHE BORE ABOUT WITH HER, SHE COULD NOT HELP KNOWING IT,
THE TORCH OF HER BEAUTY; SHE CARRIED IT ERECT INTO ANY ROOM SHE ENTERED;
AND AFTER ALL, VEIL IT AS SHE MIGHT . . . HER BEAUTY WAS APPARENT.

VIRGINIA WOOLF
English, 20th century
from *To the Lighthouse*

Nature supplies all the ingredients your body needs to be beautiful. Natural ingredients closely mirror the body's own chemistry, so they are gentle and effective. When I was a young girl, I loved making natural beauty treatments at home. When I became a model and actress, taking care of myself became a professional necessity. I researched all I could about natural beauty treatments, nutrition, fitness, aromatherapy, and meditation. My work took me all over the world, and I was exposed to many different types of people and cultures. Often when a shoot was over and the crew was heading home, I stayed on an extra week to visit the surrounding country. I was particularly intrigued by indigenous peoples and their ever-present connection with, and respect for, nature. In college, I took courses in cultural anthropology. These interests led me to join several conservation groups dedicated to preserving the unspoiled places of the world. Learning all I could about sustainable ingredients, I created a line of bath and body products (Borneo Basics) that promote sustainable use of the rainforest.

Part of the proceeds from the sale of this book will go to Conservation International, which believes that the earth's natural heritage must be maintained if future generations are to thrive spiritually, culturally, and economically. Its mission is to conserve the earth's living heritage and our global biodiversity, and to demonstrate that human societies are able to live harmoniously with nature.

This book is also dedicated to the fight against breast cancer. Part of the proceeds will be donated to Women At Risk, the Columbia-Presbyterian Medical Center's high-risk breast cancer program. The program sponsors research, education, and support services for women at high risk for developing breast cancer. It also sponsors support and educational services for women undergoing breast cancer and ovarian cancer treatment.

The recipes in this book have come from many women, including my mother, my friends, and my colleagues in the beauty industry—but they are mostly from women all over the world who use materials that are native to their regions. Naturally, none of these ingredients were tested on animals. All the ideas in this book promote the delicate balance of a woman's body, a natural extension of the balance found in the natural world.

WINKING IN THE NIGHT
THROUGH HOLES IN MY PAPER WALL-
MOON AND MILKY WAY

ISSA
Japanese, 18th century

A FEW WORDS ABOUT INGREDIENTS:

Even though something is natural, it can still be harmful. Some ingredients in these recipes, especially essential oils, are very strong, even toxic. They should never be eaten, no matter how yummy they smell. Many ingredients should not be used if you have certain medical conditions, such as high or low blood pressure or epilepsy, or are pregnant. If you are unsure about a recipe, consult your physician.

Likewise, things that are fine for you to eat can cause problems if applied externally. Before slathering a product all over your body, you should test it on a small area (the inside of your arm, or for facial products, just under your hairline) to be sure you don't have an adverse reaction. This is especially true for those with sensitive skin.

Different people experience different results. No two complexions, or heads of hair, or pairs of hands, are alike. No two people will find the same recipes and techniques equally effective. Try different recipes and give them a week or two to work. If they don't, choose something else.

Use organic ingredients whenever possible. Laboratory tests have shown that plants raised organically almost always have higher concentrations of healthful, healing substances than their conventionally grown counterparts. And besides, pesticides can be harmful and are definitely not pretty.

Many of the recipes contain only two or three ingredients. This is not merely a case of less is more; avocados, for example, are complex organisms, brimming with vitamins, minerals, and trace elements. Lavender is antiseptic and has cleansing and calming properties. Wonderful herbs, minerals, and flowers such as these are repositories of health and healing and are anything but simple.

The recipes, on the other hand, are very simple. Most of them require only a handful of ingredients and a few easy steps. Many of the ingredients are things you probably have in your kitchen right now. The rest are readily available at grocery stores, specialty markets, and health-food stores.

In fact, making up these products can and should be part of the total experience. Blending orange blossom and rose oils, mashing a juicy papaya, brewing an infusion of chamomile flowers, whipping up a honey and almond milk bath—these are sensory delights in themselves. Experiment, have fun, get messy, but don't rush. Take time to enjoy the scents and sensations of fresh fruits, exotic essences, pungent herbs.

In this hurried, harried world, quiet, contemplative time to yourself is an absolute necessity. Anxiety, frustration, tension—the recurring themes of modern life—do nothing to improve your looks. On the contrary, they release toxins into the body, inhibit circulation, and suppress the immune system. Stress can dull the most lustrous complexion, cause nails to crack and break, or turn hair brittle and lifeless. Relaxation is essential to beauty.

These products and processes don't work overnight; they work over time because they work in harmony with your body's natural chemistry. They have been passed down from generation to generation, by women who had strong ties to nature and intimate knowledge of nature's ways. These time-tested recipes and techniques promote beauty precisely because they connect you to the natural world, where your body is most at home and at ease.

THERE ARE MORE IMPORTANT THINGS TO DISCOVER IN LIFE THAN HOW TO SPEED IT UP.
MOHANDAS KARAMCHAND (MAHATMA) GANDHI
Indian, 19th to 20th century

The recipes in this book use only natural ingredients and should be safe for everyone, but skin types and body composition vary from person to person. The author and publisher cannot accept responsibility for any problems that arise in using these recipes. If you suspect you may have an adverse reaction to any of the ingredients listed, consult a physician. Before using any of the recipes, please read the reminders below.

1. Before applying any recipe or treatment to your skin, test it on a small area to be sure you have no adverse reaction. This is especially true if you have sensitive skin. Dab a little on your forearm first. Even though you may be able to eat a particular fruit or vegetable, it can still cause an allergic reaction when applied to your skin. It is always best to test, and be safe.

2. Make treatments in small quantities and keep them in the refrigerator. Unlike store-bought brands that are loaded with sometimes harmful chemical life-extenders, these products can lose their freshness in a few days if left at room temperature. Most will keep in the refrigerator for up to a week. If the ingredients separate, just process them again in a blender or stir the mixture.

3. Always make sure the bottles and jars you use to prepare and store the mixtures are clean, and wash your hands thoroughly before handling cosmetics.

4. Labeling is important. Include the name of the recipe and the date it was made (you don't want someone mistaking your facial mask for guacamole.)

5. Using a recipe once and expecting miracles is not realistic. Experiment and see what works best for your skin, since every women is different and has different needs.

6. Chapter five offers a selection of relaxation techniques and alternative methods for beating stress, but they should not be substituted for medical care. Always seek medical advice if you have a health problem.

Here are some common kitchen utensils you will need.
Most of these you probably have on hand already.

measuring cups and spoons
glass and ceramic bowls
funnel
strainer
mixing bowls
spatulas
blender or food processor
pestle and mortar
small bottles
spray bottle
(small ones specifically for the face
are available in many drug stores,
or a plant mister will do)
glass jars with lids
double boiler
small, wide frying pan
labels

Chapter One

THE FACE

The beauty of nature lies in its infinite variety and abundance. Every face is different, every face is beautiful. Every woman is a creature of nature, at once individual and special. And every woman, at any age, regardless of how well she has taken care of her skin in the past, has the potential to achieve a glowing, healthy natural beauty.

The difference is using face-care products made of natural substances. Skin, the epidermis, is the body's largest ingestive organ; all told, it weighs about nine pounds. Many creatures, such as frogs, actually breathe through their skin.

The epidermis protects us from the elements and is a major part of our immune system. It also regulates the body's natural cooling and heating system. Over time, some topical substances can be absorbed internally. That's why it is so important to ensure that anything you put on your face will not be harmful running through your blood stream.

This chapter features homemade beauty treatments made from natural ingredients that have been tested over time by women around the world. Most women will find these products

16

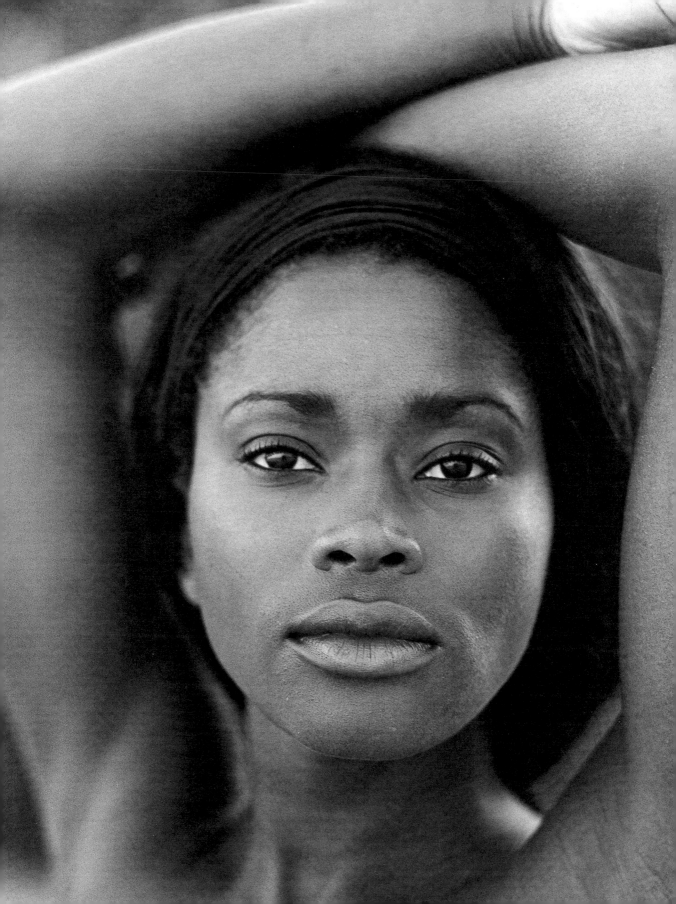

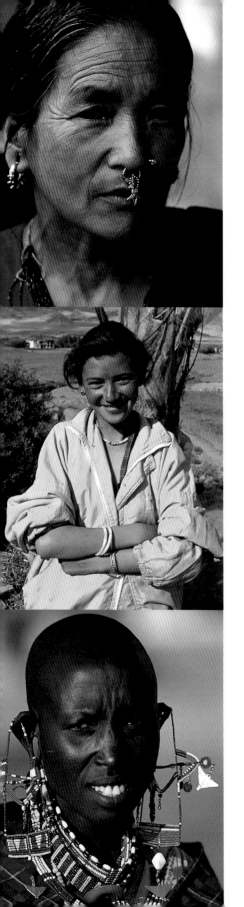

safe and effective. Equally important, not only do they save our own skin, but using these natural complexion enhancers can also help preserve our planet. It's a simple, self-evident axiom: If something is bad for the planet, it cannot be good for your face. And what's good for you is good for the environment. For instance, when you use organic ingredients, you are encouraging farmers to respect the land and water they use.

People should be beautiful in every way—
in their faces, in the way they dress,
in their thoughts and in their innermost selves.

ANTON CHEKHOV
Russian, 19th century
from *Uncle Vanya*

Wanting to be attractive is a basic instinct. Since prehistoric times, women have devised ways to look more attractive and desirable. Likewise, men have always tried to look their best to lure the objects of their affection. Women of the earliest civilizations developed ways to protect, invigorate, and improve their complexions. For the ancient Mesopotamians, attending to personal care and cleanliness was a ritual with religious overtones. They used aromatherapy oils to freshen their faces. The Queen of Hungary invented toilet water infused with rosemary. She believed it made her skin youthful and beautiful, and by all accounts it did: she was seventy-two when a young Polish king proposed marriage to her. Swedish women have traditionally used pine needles and birch leaves in their facials to clear the skin.

Beauty is not in the face; it is a light in the heart.

KAHLIL GIBRAN
Lebanese, 19th to 20th century
from *The Prophet*

18

All the lifestyle changes brought about by modern society—water and air pollution, harsh light, stress, smoking, poor diet, lack of exercise—make their mark on your face. Therefore, to really understand how to achieve a healthy complexion, you have to approach beauty from a holistic point of view. Caring for your skin from the inside is extremely important. For example, drinking fresh vegetable and fruit juices will make your skin glow.

Lasting beauty comes from within, and how you feel about yourself is ultimately what is important. Healthy-looking skin will raise your self-esteem. A beautiful face is not about putting on makeup. Beauty is individual, personal, even spiritual. A glowing complexion is, more than anything else, a reflection of radiant health, vitality, and happiness.

For many ancient cultures, the intimate relationship between one's appearance and one's inner spirit was clear. The ancient civilizations believed that physical beauty signified a person in balance with nature. Indeed, the word cosmetics comes from the Greek *kosmetikos,* which means harmony with the universe. The Greeks believed that a balance of energy and harmony showed in the face. Today, a healthy body and a beautiful inner spirit are still the best "cosmetics" a woman can have.

It's easy to forget this in today's appearance-obsessed, media-driven world. The public is presented with a seemingly endless parade of perfect-looking people. These images establish an unreal standard of beauty, undermining the self-confidence of many women, who feel they fail to live up to that unrealistic standard.

The treatments offered in this chapter do not promise perfection. In fact, one of the main aims of this book is to delineate the difference between wanting to look really good and an unrealistic desire to look perfect. It is a desire made doubly difficult when you consider that in today's throw-away society, the idea of perfect beauty changes from year to year and season to season.

The ideal of beauty has always been evanescent, shifting from era to era. From the mystical cosmetology of the ancient Egyptians, to the extravagant makeup and creams of the noblewomen and courtesans of classical Greece, from the simple beauty regimens of prehistoric hunting societies to the elaborate ornamentation of the women of the Chinese imperial court, the notion of beauty has varied tremendously from time to time and place to place.

In Sumatra, teeth filed into sharp points are a sign of beauty. In certain parts of Africa, it is simply a person's character that makes her beautiful. The Chinese consider women with round faces very beautiful.

In many cultures throughout history, youth has been an essential—though fleeting—"requirement" of ideal beauty. Today, however, we no longer accept that at a certain age a woman is in her prime, and after that she can say goodbye to beauty. A woman can be in her prime at any age, at every age. There is beauty in intelligence and power, and in the maturity from which they're derived. At eighty-six, my grandmother is full of wisdom and life experiences—and she is very beautiful.

GIVE ME BEAUTY IN THE INWARD SOUL; MAY THE OUTWARD AND THE INWARD BE AT ONE.

SOCRATES
Greek, 5th century B.C.

Like a Natural Woman

Natural is a somewhat ambiguous term in the cosmetics industry. When a label says "natural," this may not necessarily mean what the average consumer supposes. A product labeled natural can contain substances derived from natural (as opposed to man-made) sources, but these substances may have been put through so many different processes that by the time they reach the bottle they are far removed from their original state.

"Natural" does not always mean beneficial. It has been calculated that, over a lifetime, the average woman's complexion will absorb over three pounds of chemicals from cosmetic products. For example, many soaps and shampoos contain sodium lauryl sulfate. This compound can be obtained from a natural source, like coconut, or it can be processed from petroleum. Some may argue that the former is better than the latter, but the real point is that sodium lauryl sulfate, from any source, is a known carcinogen. It's been approved for topical use, but you have to consider whether it is the best thing to put on your skin. The recipes in this chapter allow you to choose genuine, bona fide natural substances that are good for your face.

After decades of obscurity, the art of making natural beauty treatments at home is becoming popular again. Now a new generation is becoming interested in getting back to the land and developing a greater appreciation for their heritage. I met a women who had recently emigrated to the United States from Russia, and she had gorgeous skin. I asked her what her secret was and she told me about her mother's natural treatments. She was kind enough to give me the recipes, and I have included them in this chapter. She claims that her mother and grandmother, who have been using these treatments for years, have youthful, radiant skin, and after trying them myself, I believe her.

Remember, the emphasis in these simple recipes is on having fun and enjoying a stronger connection to the earth. So much of modern life separates women from the natural world, putting an added strain on all of our bodily systems, and that strain shows in our faces: when people are under stress, they often have dry and taut skin; pollution and cigarette smoke can make delicate facial skin gray and wrinkled. Even natural changes and climatic conditions can affect your skin: hormonal changes can produce spots and blemishes, and dry or humid weather can affect the complexion. Skin that has been treated with natural essential oils and botanical extracts becomes stronger and healthier over time.

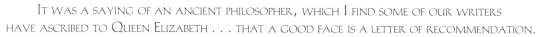

IT WAS A SAYING OF AN ANCIENT PHILOSOPHER, WHICH I FIND SOME OF OUR WRITERS
HAVE ASCRIBED TO QUEEN ELIZABETH . . . THAT A GOOD FACE IS A LETTER OF RECOMMENDATION.

JOSEPH ADDISON
English, 17th to 18th century
from *The Spectator*

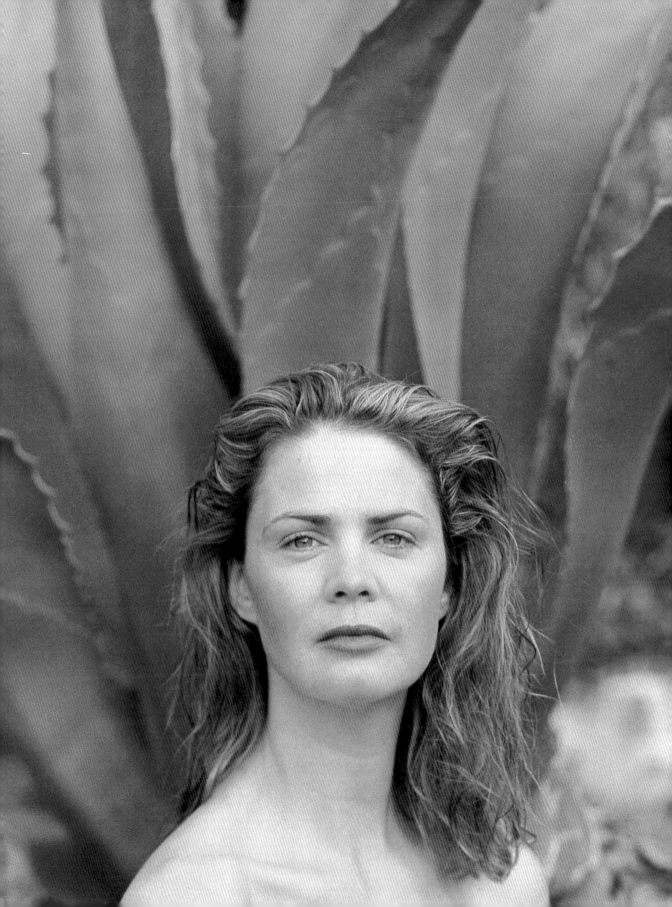

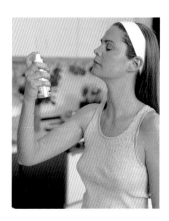

Daily Facial Care Routines

The best way to achieve a good complexion is to incorporate facial care
into your morning and evening regimen. The products in this section are gentle and
easy on your skin. They do not come with a guarantee of instant miraculous results,
but work over time as your skin begins to respond, heal, and freshen. Make preparation,
application, and enjoyment of these recipes part of your daily routine.
A good complexion comes not from triage of occasional problems—a patch of
dry skin here, that nagging blemish there—but rather it requires
constant care and nourishment, from inside out.

Morning Face Cleansing

1 Splash face with warm water
2 Cleanse face with oils or scrubs,
   depending on skin type (see recipes)
3 Rinse with warm water
4 Tone your skin with an astringent
   to clean off any residue from
   cleansers
5 Mist face with Evian
   or floral water (see recipes)
6 Moisturize

Evening Face Cleansing

1 Remove all dirt and makeup with
   natural soap (any glycerin-based soap),
   or vegetable or jojoba oil and cotton pads
2 Mix your favorite essential oil(s)
   with a little sesame oil, and give yourself
   a light massage (optional)
3 You might want to use a mask, scrub,
   or fruit peel once every week or two,
   depending on your skin type
4 Mist with Evian or floral water (see recipes)
5 Moisturize

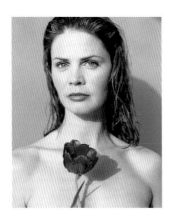

Natural Cleansers

A good, thorough cleansing should be at the heart of every morning and evening routine. This does not mean, however, that your face needs to be subjected to twice-daily doses of rigorous scrubbing with harsh chemicals. Some people are overzealous in their quest for a squeaky-clean complexion. If your skin squeaks, that probably means it has been stripped of oils essential for its good health.

Dirt, pollution, makeup, and dead skin cells have got to go. They clog pores and make skin dull and lifeless. On the other hand, overworked, over-cleansed skin also loses its luster. There are ways to get rid of the mess without messing up your complexion. Use gentle cleansers, and always finish with a moisturizer to replenish any softness stripped away with the dirt.

Soap can be very drying. Look for an all-natural, vegetable-based (not petroleum- or animal product–based) soap or glycerin soap. These soaps help keep the complexion's delicate acid-base equation in balance.

Loofahs are too harsh and rough for use on the face. It is best to use cotton pads, balls, a washcloth, or a natural sponge. Whatever you choose, make sure it's clean, and don't use anyone else's. You don't want to add extraneous bacteria to the face.

For makeup removal, use oils that are cold-pressed. This means that the oils have been extracted by a heat-free process that maintains their vitamin, enzyme, and mineral content.

Topical oils

Choose the best oils for your skin type. If you have combination skin (oily around the forehead, nose, and chin; normal to dry elsewhere) use the oils that are appropriate for each area. Remember that all these oils are free of preservatives, so they need to be refrigerated. For an explanation of what different essential oils do for the skin, see page 34.

For dry skin. Avocado, almond, olive (extra virgin), and apricot kernel oils, as well as cocoa butter, are nondrying. A light coat on fresh, clean skin won't clog pores and will seal in moisture. Regular soap for makeup removal can be very drying, so use a pure vegetable soap.

For normal to oily skin. Sesame, jojoba, safflower, corn, and sunflower oils perk up pores and leave the skin glowing, not greasy.

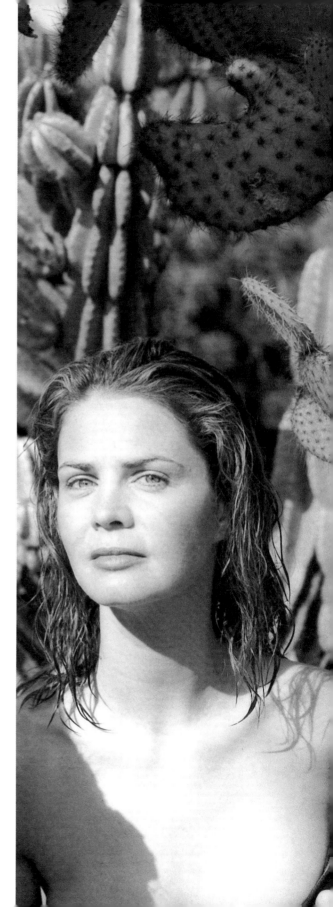

Native American Jojoba Makeup Remover

Jojoba is native to the Southwestern United States and has for centuries been prized by tribal peoples for its many soothing and healing properties. Jojoba oil is very gentle, yet will easily remove all makeup. Eye tissue is very delicate, so be careful not to rub. The under-eye area is especially fragile. Eyes are also highly susceptible to infection, so always wash your hands and use clean or sterile pads. Avoid products like Vaseline, mineral oil, and baby oil. These are petroleum-based and can clog pores and rob skin of nutrients. Always read the labels, and choose only vegetable-derived oils.

Cotton pads
Jojoba oil (found in any health food store)

Saturate two clean cotton pads in warm water. Squeeze out any excess water. Put a few drops of jojoba oil on the pads. Close your eyes and stroke the eyelids downward, finishing on the lashes. Clean one lid at a time, working from the outside corner to the inside corner. When you are finished with the eyes, moisten a few cotton pads with oil to remove makeup from the rest of your face using an upward motion. Then splash your face with lots of cool water and pat dry.

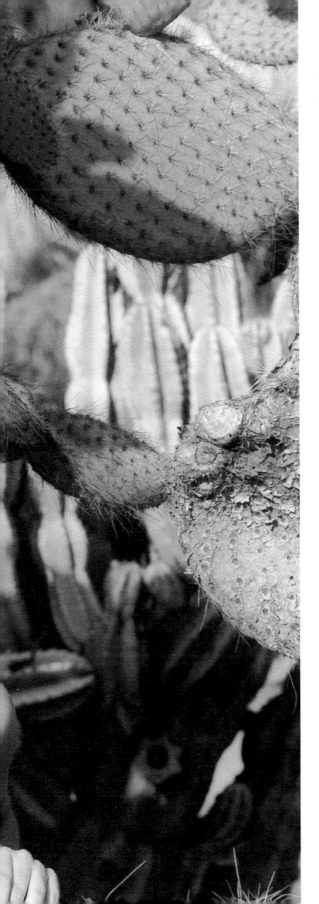

Helen of Troy Almond Cleanser

Helen's famous beauty caused as much trouble for Doctor Faustus as she did for Paris and Menelaus 2,800 years before, as recounted by poets from Homer to Yeats.

The women of the Greek aristocracy were well known for their elaborate beauty preparations. The almond is cultivated in Greece and throughout the Mediterranean, where its oil is used to soothe dry skin. Here is a recipe that Helen might have concocted to preserve her charms when whisked away to the arid plains of Troy.

1 tablespoon plain yogurt
1 teaspoon almond butter (available at health food stores) or 1 teaspoon almond oil

Mix the ingredients together and apply to your face, starting at the base of the neck and massaging gently upward in a circular motion. Remove the cleanser with dampened cotton pads or a clean washcloth.

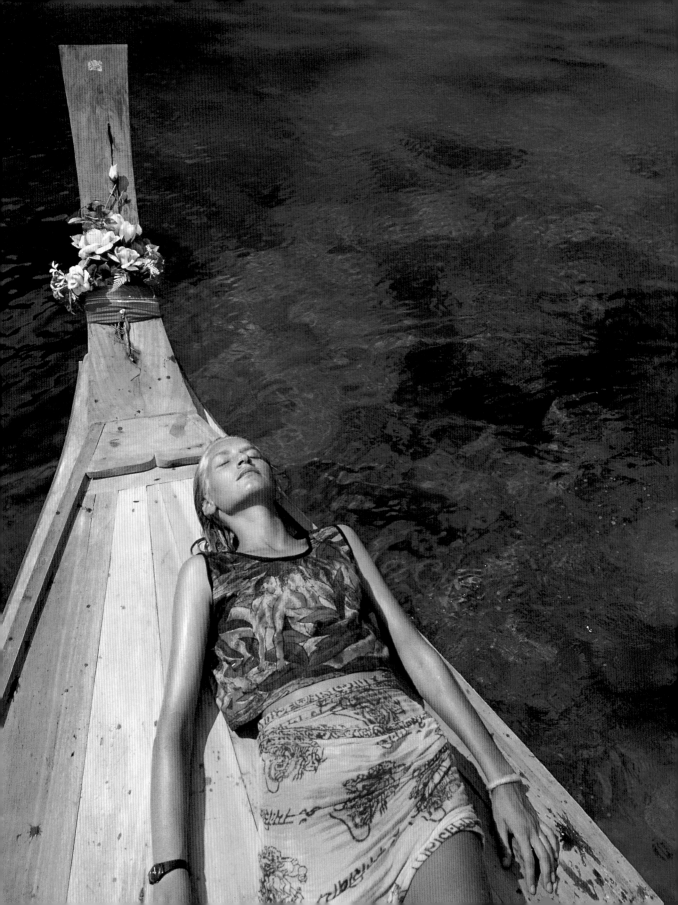

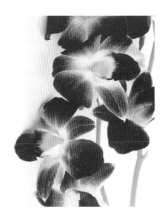

Tahitian Cocoa Butter Cleanser

The women of Tahiti are known for their gorgeous skin and hair. Cocoa butter, derived from the cocoa bean, is one of their great beauty staples; they use it to counteract the drying effects of salt air and intense sun (it acts as a natural sunscreen). Cocoa butter is especially nourishing to skin during extreme weather conditions that dry the skin in winter and summer.

1 to 4 tablespoons cocoa butter
1/2 cup avocado or almond oil
1 to 2 tablespoons soya margarine

Place the cocoa butter, oil, and margarine in a double boiler. Melt the ingredients over low heat, stirring until they are thoroughly blended. Remove from the heat and beat with an electric blender or a whisk until the cleanser is cooled. Place in a jar and label. This effective cleansing cream can be applied all over the body, especially on dry areas.

Mila's Soothing Sunburn Remedy

My friend Mila, an actress and producer, goes back to her Slavic roots to battle stress herbally, using herbs that are indigenous to her father's countryside. This wonderful Slavic herbal remedy will also soothe sunburn.

2 heaping tablespoons St. John's Wort leaves
8-10 ounce spray bottle of safflower oil

Add a few heaping tablespoons of St. John's Wort leaves to a spray bottle of safflower oil. Leave it on the windowsill exposed to the sun for a week. Apply to sunburn for soothing relief.

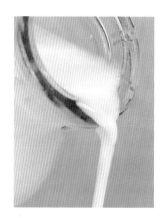

Buttermilk & Lemon Cleanser

This rich concoction is perfect for oily skin. Buttermilk acts as a bleach for sunspots or freckles. The lemon acts as a toning agent, and the combination with the buttermilk is bracing and refreshing.

1 to 3 tablespoons buttermilk
1 to 3 teaspoons lemon juice
1 to 3 tablespoons yogurt (optional)

Whisk the ingredients together.
Place in a clean jar, label, and refrigerate.
Apply to face and neck, then wipe off with cotton pads.

Frightfully English Light Milk Cleansers

These cleansers remind me of the flavors of a proper English afternoon tea: fresh cucumber sandwiches and heaps of strawberries and cream. Strawberries and cucumbers have astringent qualities and are excellent cleansers.

1/4 to 1/2 cup strawberries or peeled, seeded, and chopped cucumber
1/4 to 1/2 pint whole milk

In an electric blender combine the strawberries or the cucumbers with the milk. Let steep for a few hours. Shake well.
Place in a clean bottle, label, and refrigerate.
Because base solutions are light, use a cotton pad to apply to the face, then rinse.

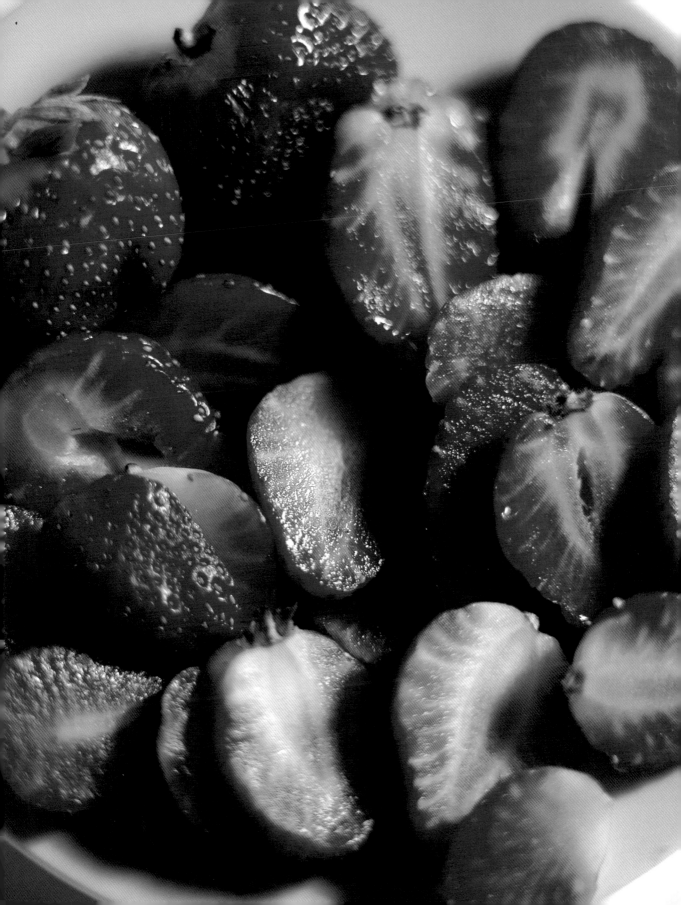

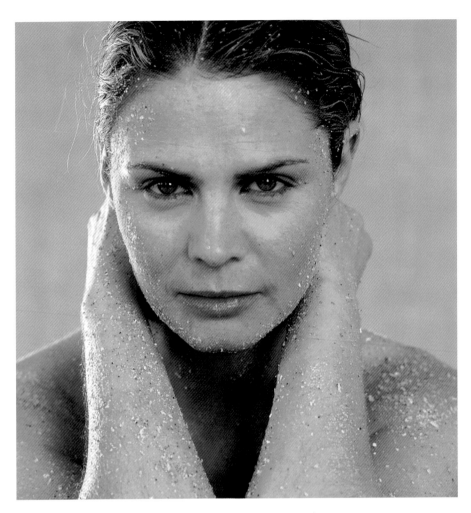

Face Cleansers: Scrubs

Most women, at certain times, suffer from a complexion that is dull and lifeless. This often occurs because the face is covered by a thin layer of built-up dirt, oils, and dead skin cells. Exfoliants have become wildly popular in the last few years; you can find them in everything from lip balms to bikini wax preparations. Actually, women have known about the beneficial properties of exfoliants for centuries. These substances help the complexion to renew itself by sloughing off dead skin cells at a faster-than-normal rate. Oatmeal, bran, cornmeal, almond meal, and Wheatena brand cereal are great cleansers that also have exfoliating properties. They are gentle, inexpensive, and quick and easy to use. Keep a small covered jar of any of these in your bathroom. Just mix with a little water or witch hazel.

All the following recipes are mild; however, it's best to test their effects on your complexion in a small area before use. People with very sensitive skin or extremely dry skin may want to avoid scrubs.

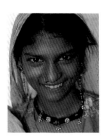

Healing Honey Cleanser

Honey has been used for centuries by beauty-conscious women as a natural cosmetic. It's a great facial cleanser as well as a nourisher and healer. Colombian women use honey as a mask. It is also a natural humectant, or skin softener. Wheat germ is antiseptic and toning. This is a good treatment for blemishes.

1 to 2 tablespoons honey
1 teaspoon wheat germ,
for blemishes

Combine the honey and wheat germ, if using. Moisten your face with a little warm water. Dab the mixture on lightly with fingers or apply directly to blemishes with a cotton swab. Leave on for 15 to 30 minutes. Rinse off with warm water.

Yogi Yogurt Cleanser

This is a wonderful cleanser for people with oily or normal skin. If you have dry skin, simply puncture a vitamin E capsule and mix it into the yogurt and omit the salt. Yogurt is loaded with protein, calcium, and vitamins and is a very soothing cleanser.

1 to 3 tablespoons yogurt
Pinch of salt

Combine the yogurt and salt.
Slather the mixture onto your face.
Rinse off with tepid water.

Bombay Cleanser

While traveling through certain parts of India, I noticed that a form of cornmeal was used by the women to scrub and wash the face. Oatmeal is nourishing to the skin and is used in many parts of the world as a beauty aid.

1 to 2 tablespoons oatmeal
(or colloidal oatmeal)
1 to 2 teaspoons witch hazel
A few drops of water

Dampen the oatmeal, then add the witch hazel and a few drops of water to make it moist. Apply to face with an upward and outward circular motion. Splash with lots of warm water to remove all surface dirt. This recipe can be adapted for all skin types; if your skin is extra dry, add a little vegetable oil to the mixture. You can also make this recipe into a nourishing mask by adding a mashed banana.

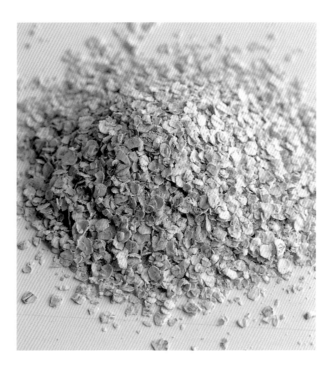

Sow Your Oats
Cleansing Scrub

Colloidal oatmeal dissolves easily and always leaves the skin feeling silky and smooth. It's very soothing and is often prescribed for itchy skin conditions like chicken pox.

1 teaspoon colloidal oatmeal
(or ground almonds)
1 teaspoon honey
1 teaspoon yogurt
1/2 teaspoon sea salt
1/2 teaspoon almond oil
(optional, for dry skin)

Combine all the ingredients together in a ceramic bowl and apply to a clean face. Massage gently into your skin with an upward, outward circular motion. Then splash your face several times with tepid water.

John O'Groats Oats
Blemish Cleanser

Oats have long been a staple in the Scottish diet: in oatmeal, oatcakes, whiskey, and ale. Caledonian custom has it that oats placed in the newlyweds' pantry will ensure a happy and fruitful marriage. This mixture is great for blemished skin. Lemon juice is an antiseptic and cleanser that restores acidity to the skin.

3 tablespoons colloidal oatmeal
1 teaspoon unprocessed honey
1/4 cup warm water
1 teaspoon white wine vinegar
1 teaspoon freshly squeezed lemon juice

Combine the ingredients to form a paste. Apply to a clean face, massaging gently into the skin. You can leave it on for up to 5 minutes, then rinse with warm water.

Most ancient civilizations used some form of aromatherapy. Incense was an essential part of ritual from prehistoric times and continues in modern-day religious ceremonies throughout the world. Both an ancient art and a science, aromatherapy restores harmony between mind, body, and spirit.

Frankincense was precious to the ancient world. Its vapor was believed to elevate the spirit. In ancient Greece, Athenian ladies would burn powdered myrrh to penetrate the face and act as a healing astringent. The emperors of ancient Persia would fill the streams that ran through their gardens with the fragrant essence of rose.

Many people are rediscovering aromatherapy as a natural means to restore harmony between mind and body. Aromatherapy is widely practiced in Europe as a healing technique. In England, midwives prescribe warm lavender baths to help soothe and relax women during labor.

These oils are highly concentrated, and hence very potent. When using essential oils for skin care, always be sure they are at a low concentration—that is, highly diluted with carrier oils.

Carrier Oils

Carrier oils are used to dilute essential oils. Use a carrier oil any time you want to apply an essential oil directly to your skin. Because essential oils are so concentrated, you need to add only a few drops.

The following carrier oils contain minerals, vitamins, and protein and are good for all skin types. Any you can't find at the supermarket should be available at health-food stores:

jojoba oil	safflower oil
almond oil	avocado oil
grapeseed oil	sunflower oil
sweet almond oil	sesame oil

Mixing Oils

It is best to mix oils in a clean glass container or glass bottle. Use a separate dropper for each essential oil. Many oils are light sensitive and will lose potency if exposed to the sun. Herbalists, therefore, prefer storing oils in indigo, brown, or other dark-colored glass containers.

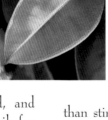

Essential oils evaporate on contact with air, so to combine them it is best to shake them in a closed container, rather than stirring them in a bowl. Add four or five drops of each essential oil to the bottle. Shake the bottle to mix, and test the effect and fragrance. Experiment. You might want to use one or a few essential oils. When you find a scent you like, add about eight ounces of the carrier oil. Keep a log of the number of drops you use of the essential oils in your blend, so you can reproduce it. You can also note the therapeutic effects and your experience of the fragrance. Custom-blend oils for friends. They make wonderful gifts.

Oils for Normal & General Skincare:

GERANIUM

LAVENDER

LEMON

YLANG-YLANG

CHAMOMILE

JASMINE

SANDALWOOD

ROSE

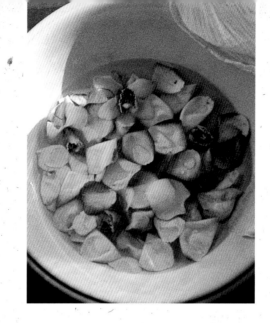

Oils for Oily Skin:

GERANIUM

LEMON

BASIL

YLANG-YLANG

WITCH HAZEL

FRANKINCENSE

GRAPEFRUIT

PEPPERMINT

Oils for Dry Skin:

ROSEMARY

CARROT SEED

JASMINE

SANDALWOOD

ROSE

OLIVE

CHAMOMILE

Oils for Rough, Distressed Skin:

JOJOBA

ALOE

ALMOND

COMFREY ROOT

Oils for Sensitive Skin:

CHAMOMILE

ROSE

NEROLI

LAVENDER

ORANGE BLOSSOM

Oils for Wrinkled Skin:

PALMAROSA

CARROT SEED

MYRRH

Oils for Blemished Skin:

TEA TREE

JUNIPER

BERGAMOT

LAVENDER

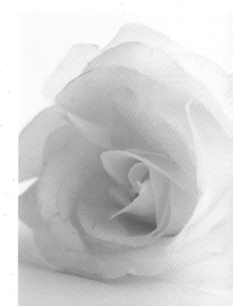

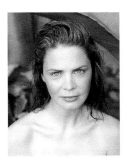

NANCY SPRAGUE'S MORNING FACE MASSAGE

Nancy is a friend and a prominent makeup artist.
She showed me how to do this quick, self-nurturing face massage with essential oils.

1 Warm the skin. I often do this by steaming. I prepare a bowl of boiling water and dried flowers—either roses, which have a purifying effect, or chamomile (you can just open the tea bags and pour the contents into the boiling water), which acts as an anti-inflammatory. You can also use lavender, which can stimulate circulation and help if you're feeling irritable, or eucalyptus, which acts as a decongestant and can help you overcome sluggishness. Or you could add a few drops of Neroli or orange blossom—one of my favorites. After adding the flowers to the boiling water, I hold my head several inches above for five minutes, using a towel over my head to hold the steam in. If I can't steam my face or I am giving the facial massage to someone else, I soak a clean white towel in the infused water. After removing it, I let it cool and hold it against the face for five minutes.

2 Mix a few teaspoons of a carrier oil such as sweet almond oil with 1 to 2 drops of essential oil.

3 Rub mixture in hands to warm.

4 Cup your hands over your face and inhale the essential oils. Let the calming effects soothe you.

5 Gently spread your hands across your face moving toward your temples.

6 Gently press the sides of your thumb against your upper eyelid and apply momentary pressure.

7 Follow the eye socket outward and then around to just above the center of the cheek, stopping to apply pressure at each point. This will help to relieve water retention around the eyes.

8 With the five fingers of each hand, apply pressure to the temples.

9 Criss-cross fingers on the forehead.

10 Work upward from the neck, moving up the face into the hair. Always use upward and outward strokes.

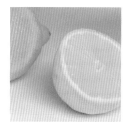

Fruits:

    mango
    orange
    apple
    papaya
    pear
    pineapple
    tomato
    grape
    lemon
    grapefruit

Liquids:

    aged milk
    buttermilk
    yogurt

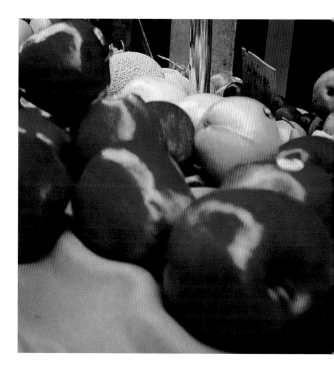

Alpha-Hydroxy Acid: Fruit Peels

Alpha-hydroxy acids or AHAs are a buzzword in the world of exfoliants.
Like most "discoveries," AHAs, in one form or other, have actually been used for centuries by such famous beauties as Cleopatra, whose flawless skin has been attributed to her passion for milk baths. The gentle exfoliation of these fruit peels speeds up cell renewal, leading to a healthier skin tone. You can try one of these ingredients, or mix and match with the liquids to find a formula that best suits your skin. These peels contain organic acids and can be used to help soften the appearance of wrinkles; minimize sun spots, age spots, and blemishes; and unclog pores. Do not expect miracles right away. Over time you will notice a difference.
Make sure to test a small area first before applying to your whole face.

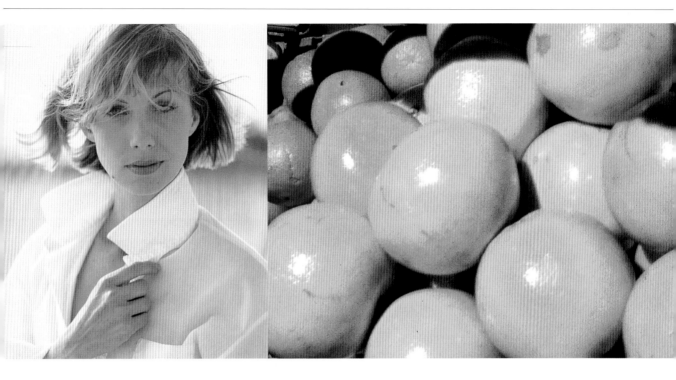

There are two ways to apply these peels. The simplest is straight from the fruit. Peel, pit, or core, and mash the fruit; then either slather the pulp over your face or massage the juice into your skin. Leave on for about 10 minutes. Papaya juice should be left on for no more than 5 minutes. To refresh tired-looking skin, try cutting pineapple into slices and placing them directly on your face. Leave on for 5 to 10 minutes then splash with cool water.

You can also make a fruit-peel mask, by adding 1 to 2 tablespoons clay to the mashed fruit. Slather the mixture on your face and leave on for about 15 minutes before rinsing. If your skin is dry, add a few drops of honey or vegetable oil to any of these mixtures.

Cleopatra's Milk Face Lift

1/2 cup whole or aged milk

The butterfat in milk will nourish and soften the skin. The lactic acid found in fermented milk is a great beauty enhancer. Apply the whole milk to wrinkles and eyelids, wait 5 to 10 minutes, then rinse off. Repeat often to smooth out wrinkles and creases around the eyes. If your skin is sensitive, do not apply to your entire face.

Take the breath of the new dawn
And make it part of you.
It will give you strength.
Hopi saying

Toners

A toner is used after cleansing to remove oil and residue. A toner closes pores, replacing the protective acid mantle that preserves the skin's proper pH and guards against infection.

For dry skin, use aloe vera. Mist the face often during the day. Avoid products that contain witch hazel, alcohol, or citrus as the primary ingredient. Avoid heavy scrubs.

For oily skin, use witch hazel, or citrus extracts.
Apply on oily areas only, not all over the face.

For normal skin, try any of the toners below.

Mashed Cucumber Toner

Cucumber was considered a delicacy by the Ancient Egyptians, Greeks, and Romans. Women of Martinique slice and squeeze fresh cucumbers to extract the juice and use it directly on the skin. It is thought that cucumbers contain elements that may prevent wrinkles. They close pores and are cleansing and refreshing.

1 peeled, seeded, and mashed cucumber
1/2 teaspoon honey

Put the ingredients in an electric blender, and blend until smooth. Bottle, label, and refrigerate. Apply with a cotton pad.

Pioneer Spirit Toner

Western tribes taught the early pioneers how to boil the leaves and bark of the herb witch hazel, a plant that Native Americans used for divining rods, as well as for reducing swelling from wounds, on muscle aches, inflammation, and bruises. Yogurt is cleansing and has a gentle bleaching action that works to lighten dark spots and age spots, evening out skin tones.

1 teaspoon witch hazel
1 egg white, lightly beaten
1 peeled, mashed cucumber
1 teaspoon rosewater (or distilled water)
1/2 teaspoon honey
1 to 2 teaspoons plain yogurt (optional)

Put the ingredients in an electric blender, and blend until smooth. Bottle, label, and refrigerate. Apply with a cotton pad. You can leave the toner on, or rinse it off with warm water.

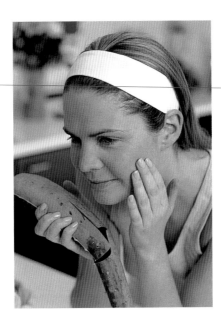

Egyptian Queen Toner

(for oily skin)

The *Papyrus Ebers,* an Egyptian document written around 1500 B.C., records the use of aloe in many different areas, from cooking to cosmetics. It is excellent for all kinds of skin problems, especially burns, cuts, and rashes.

1/2 cup pure aloe juice or gel (not synthetic)
1/2 cup cucumber juice
Juice of 1/2 lemon

Put the ingredients in a container with a tight lid. Shake until thoroughly blended. Bottle, label, and refrigerate. Shake well before each use. Dampen a cotton pad with the liquid and apply to your face and neck. You can leave the toner on or rinse it off with warm water.

Russian Fruit Toner

(for oily skin)

Vodka means "water of life" in Slavic languages, and is of course a favorite libation in Russia. It also a makes a great toner for complexions dulled by pollution, wind, and cold. Grapefruit is great for oily skin, helping to balance overactive oil glands.

1/2 cup grapefruit juice
1/2 teaspoon lemon juice
1/2 teaspoon vodka
 1 teaspoon water

Put the ingredients in a container with a tight lid. Shake until thoroughly blended. Bottle, label, and refrigerate. Shake well before each use. Dampen a cotton pad with the liquid and apply to your face and neck. You can leave the toner on or rinse it off with warm water.

Toners for Different Skin Types

For oily or blemished skin:

·Add 3 parts aloe juice to 1 part water;
put in a spray bottle and spritz
all over your face.

·Add 2 ounces apple juice to 2
ounces lemon juice; dab on your face
with a cotton pad.

·Mash fresh cucumber,
tomato, grapefruit,
lemon, apple, or strawberries;
gently rub all over your face.
Then rinse off with tepid water.

For dry skin:

·Mix equal parts aloe juice
and purified sea water
(available at health-food stores);
put in a spray bottle and spritz all
over your face.

·Dilute 4 ounces papaya juice
with 1/2 teaspoon lemon juice;
gently rub or massage all over
your face. Then rinse off.

·Rub face with mashed peach, pear,
or cantaloupe. Then rinse off.

·Add a little vitamin E or evening
primrose oil to a quarter-sized dab of
aloe gel; massage into your face.

For all skin types:

·Apple cider vinegar is excellent for
dry, flaky skin and can be used
straight from the bottle on a
cotton pad, or poured into a bath.

·Add a few drops of apple cider vinegar
to 4 ounces distilled or mineral water;
put in a spray bottle and spritz
all over your face.

·Egg white is an astringent
and can be applied to your face
with a cotton pad.
Always rinse off.

·Witch hazel can be applied to your
face with a cotton pad.

For normal skin:

·Use any of the above toners.

·Mix equal parts
aloe juice and distilled
or mineral water;
put in a spray bottle
and spritz all
over your face.

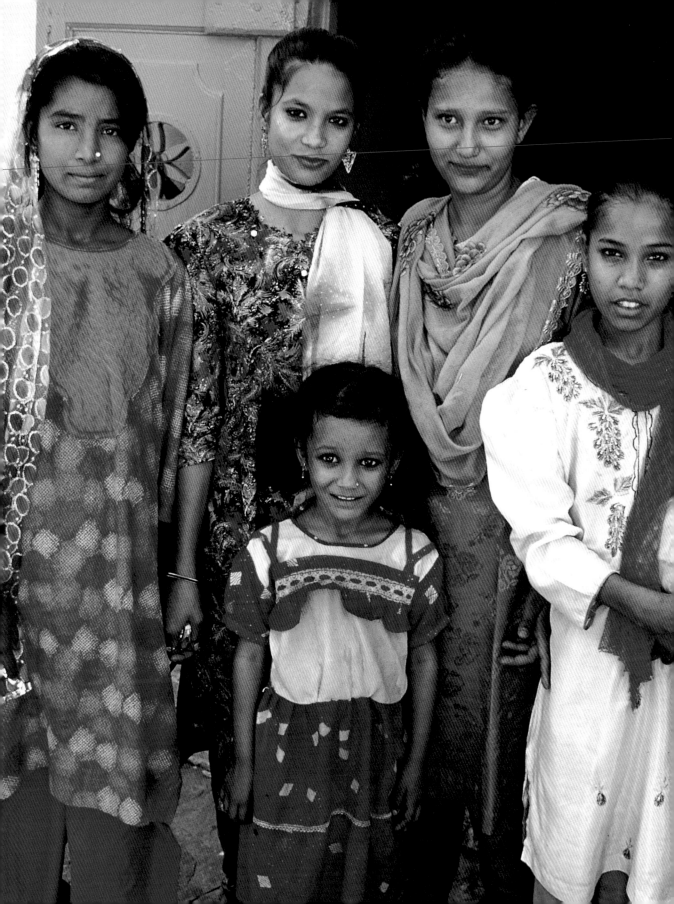

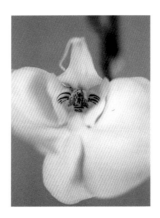

Floral Waters

Water has cleansing, healing, and restorative properties. Mist your face and neck regularly to replenish moisture lost during the day due to sun, dry heat, stress, and pollution. Evian makes a great mineral water spray, or you can make your own. A mixture of aloe vera juice and mineral water or distilled water is very healing and moisturizing. You can make your floral waters astringent by adding witch hazel or juices and cutting back on the water. Always keep floral waters refrigerated. Allow the water to dry naturally, and do not blot dry. Test your spray on a small area before using.

Rose water: 1 cup distilled water and 1 ounce crushed rose buds or petals
Orange water: 1 cup distilled water and 1 ounce crushed orange flowers
Lavender water: 1 cup distilled water and 1 ounce lavender flowers

Combine the ingredients in a spray or flip-top bottle. Spray directly onto the face or dampen a cotton pad and dab on.

Morning Floral Spritz

This is the easiest way to use essential oils on the skin, and is a freshening energizer in the morning or any time you need a pick-me-up.

5 to 8 drops essential floral oils such as rose, lavender, chamomile, or geranium
4 ounces distilled water

Combine the ingredients in a spray bottle. Shake well before use.

Tea Time Spritz

1 to 2 bags herbal tea
such as chamomile, ginseng,
or rosehips (high in vitamin C),
alone or in any combination you like

Brew the tea to medium strength,
let cool, strain, and put in
a spray bottle or clean
perfume atomizer.

Citrusy Spritz

This works well for oily and/or blemished skin. The grapefruit helps regulate overactive oil glands. The rosemary helps with trouble spots like blemishes. The smell is wonderful and refreshing.

4 ounces distilled water
1 drop lime oil
1 drop grapefruit oil
1 drop lemon oil
1 drop rosemary oil

Combine the ingredients in a spray bottle. Shake well before use.

THE LIGHT OF LOVE, THE PURITY OF GRACE,
THE MIND, THE MUSIC BREATHING FROM HER FACE,
THE HEART WHOSE SOFTNESS HARMONIZED THE WHOLE
AND, OH! THAT EYE WAS IN ITSELF A SOUL!

LORD BYRON
English, 19th century
from *The Bride of Abydos*

SOLUTIONS FOR PUFFY EYES

My mother taught me that moist tea bags work wonders. With your eyes closed, place a moistened, warm (not hot) tea bag on each eyelid. You can use a regular black tea or a chamomile tea bag. You can also take several chamomile tea bags, moisten them in cold water and refrigerate them. If you wake up with swollen or puffy eyes, just apply a chilled bag to your eyes.

- A slice of cucumber on each eye is refreshing.
- Slices of cucumber soaked in milk combat puffiness.
- Slices of potato wrapped in gauze work well on puffy eyes.
- Cotton pads or balls soaked in cold milk will deflate puffy areas.
- Cotton pads or balls soaked in witch hazel and left on your eyelids for 10 minutes relieve puffiness, eye fatigue, and eye strain.
- A stiffly beaten egg white applied to the face or under the eyes with a brush will reduce puffiness. You can add a few drops of witch hazel, which also reduces swelling, to help keep the egg white from drying too quickly.

- With your eyes open, soak your face for a minute or two in a bowl of cold distilled water.
- Use a humidifier in winter when rooms are dry and overheated, or fill a pan with water and place on the radiator to keep moisture in the air.
- Take GLA (gamma-linolenic acid), like flaxseed oil, evening primrose oil, or borage oil internally. Any of these oils can act as anti-inflammatories.
- For red eyes, try eyebright tea, made with the eyebright herb.
- Get plenty of sleep. For most people, at least eight hours per night.

STEAM HEAT

Treating yourself to an herb-infused steam or an infusion of essential oils is an excellent method of cleansing the skin and treating blemishes (see page 60 for box on how to give yourself a facial). You can steam your face weekly to triage troubled skin, or monthly for normal maintenance. There are many benefits to steaming:

1 Deep cleans the pores and helps eliminate toxins;
2 Cleanses the skin of surface dirt and grime;
3 Increases blood circulation; and
4 Softens lines and helps hydrate the skin.

One of the beauties of steaming is its simplicity. Put dried herbs or tea bags in a large heat-proof bowl and cover with boiling water. Create a tent by wrapping a towel around your head and draping it over the outer rim of the bowl. Hold your face about 12 inches from the bowl. Close your eyes and enjoy the relaxing steam, letting the cares of the day slip away. Allow the steam to penetrate your face for about 10 to 15 minutes for oily skin, about 3 to 5 minutes for dry skin. After steaming, splash on cold water, and pat dry with a towel.

When using essential oils instead of dried herbs or teas, let the water cool a little before adding 3 to 5 drops of essential oil, so that the oils won't evaporate too quickly. For normal skin, try chamomile oil. For oily skin, try peppermint oil. For dry skin, try rosemary or sandalwood oil.

People with sensitive skin or small blood capillaries that look like tiny hair-like veins should never use hot masks or hot facials. Seek professional beauty therapy advice.

Chamomile Steam

(for normal or dry skin)

2 drops chamomile oil
2 to 3 drops rosemary oil

Pour boiling water into a heat-proof bowl. Let it sit until it is still hot, but no longer boiling, then add the oils.

Peppermint Steam

(for normal or oily skin)

2 drops peppermint oil
3 drops geranium oil

Pour boiling water into a heat-proof bowl. Let sit until it is still hot, but no longer boiling, then add the oils.

Papaya Steam (for normal skin)

2 papaya or papaya-mint tea bags (available at health-food stores)

Place the tea bags in a heat-proof bowl, and add almost-boiling water.

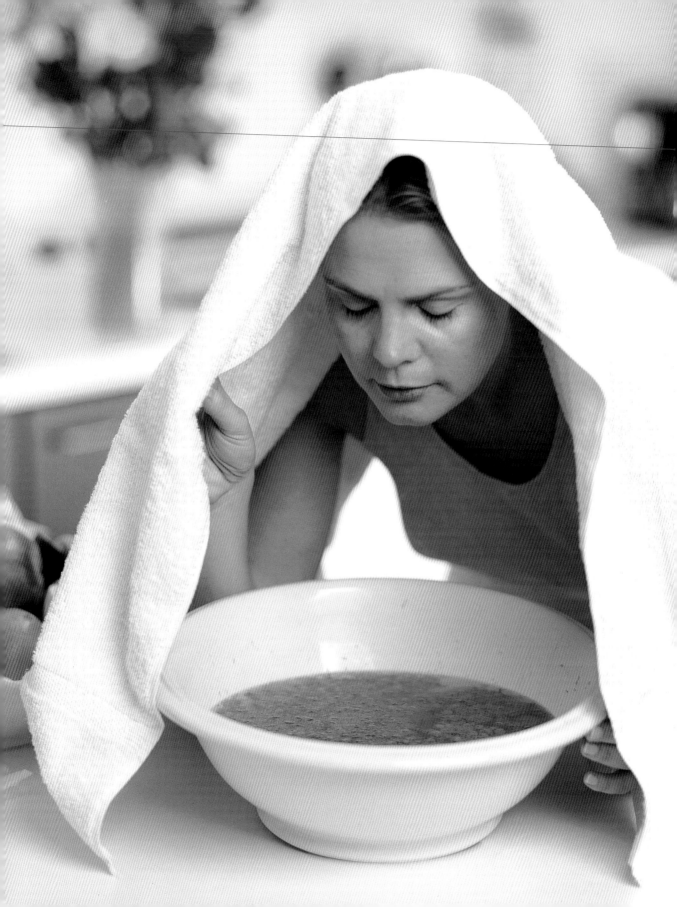

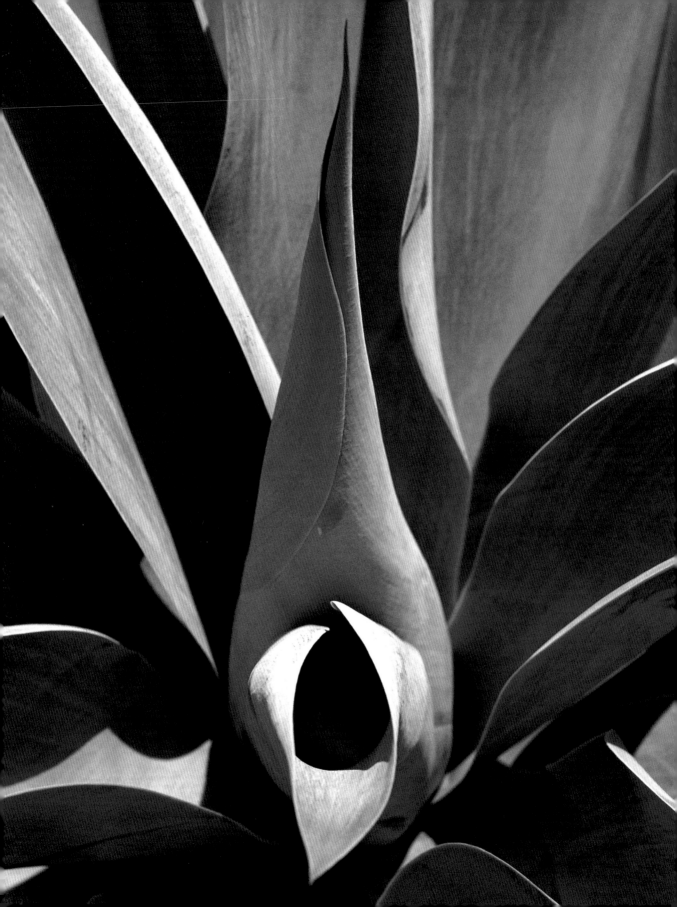

MOISTURIZERS

Moisturizing your face regularly is extremely important. It's the final step in a facial routine, giving the complexion a healthy finish by replenishing elements stripped away by pollution, sun, wind, and cleansers. It helps restore vitality and keeps skin in balance.

Honey After-Bath Lotion

1 tablespoon honey
1/2 cup cold water
A few drops apple cider vinegar

Combine all the ingredients and apply all over your face and neck right after your bath or shower. Let dry naturally and leave on or rinse off. Honey will moisturize and soften your skin.

Revitalizing Moisturizer

This wonderful combination of oils will do wonders for your skin. The oils will absorb into your skin, leaving it soft and moist. The healing oils of vitamin A and E, and primrose oil give skin the nutrients it needs.

1 tablespoon olive oil
2 tablespoons avocado oil
2 tablespoons almond oil
2 tablespoons sesame oil
2 to 5 capsules vitamin E oil (400 I.U.)
2 capsules vitamin A (50,000 I.U.)
2 to 5 capsules evening primrose oil (optional)
2 to 3 drops lavender, ylang-ylang, or geranium essential oil (optional)

Pour the avocado, almond, olive, and sesame oils into a dark bottle or small jar. Prick the capsules with a pin or cut them with scissors, and empty into the bottle with the base oils. Add an essential oil and shake well. Take a quarter-sized dab in your hand, and massage gently into your face, neck, and hands. The moisturizer can occasionally be left on overnight, but don't overdo it—skin needs to breathe freely while you sleep. All these oils are stable, so you can double the recipe if you like, label the bottle, and save the extra in the refrigerator. Shake well before using.

Quickie Moisturizers

These simple recipes are perfect for the gal on the go who wants to get gorgeous.

· Combine glycerine and rosewater.
· Mix almond oil with a drop of honey and peach juice.
· Prick a capsule of vitamin E and smear the oil all over your face.
· Olive oil, almond oil, and avocado oil are wonderful penetrating oils for the skin. Add a few drops of lavender or ylang-ylang essential oils and massage into your face.

Pampering Rose Moisturizer

1 to 2 teaspoons jojoba oil
1 to 3 teaspoons sweet almond oil
2 drops rose essential oil (optional)
1 to 2 drops jasmine or lavender oil

Combine the jojoba oil and sweet almond oil to make a base oil. Combine the essential oils, and then add to the base oil. You can experiment with your favorite essential oils, depending on your skin type. Remember, just a few drops go a long way. With clean hands, smooth the moisturizing oil all over your face, neck, and shoulders. (See Nancy Sprague's Morning Face Massage on page 35 for application instructions.)

Maharani Sandalwood Moisturizer

Sandalwood comes from the roots of an evergreen tree native to India and Indonesia. Sandalwood incense is often used as an aid to meditation in India. This oil, with its sexy, woodsy aroma, is great for dry skin. Jojoba and avocado are nourishing and soothing.

3 teaspoons jojoba oil
2 teaspoons avocado oil
2 drops sandalwood oil
1 drop rosemary oil
1 drop jasmine or carrot seed oil

Combine the sandalwood, rosemary, and jasmine oil, and then add the jojoba and avocado oils. (See Nancy Sprague's Morning Face Massage on page 35 for application instructions.)

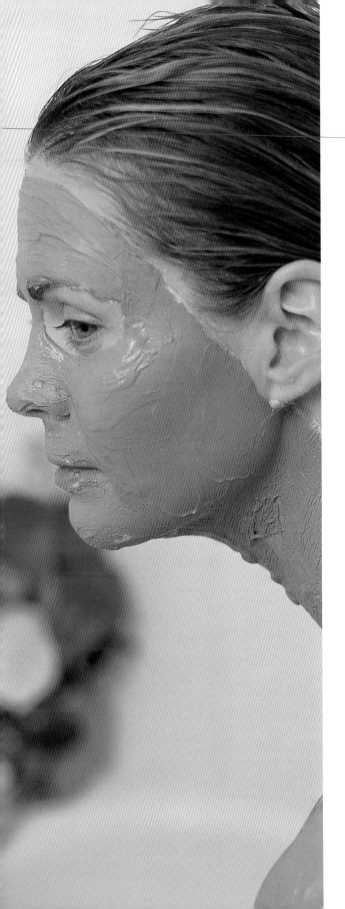

Masks and Treatments

Women have been using masks of mud and clay for thousands of years to brighten dull, lifeless skin. These recipes are wonderful for giving the skin a feeling of freshness and renewal.

Juniper Soothing Oil for Blemishes

Juniper is a favorite among herbalists—virtually all parts of the plant are useful. Juice from the berries is antiseptic and contains an antibiotic.

4 teaspoons olive oil
1 to 3 drops juniper oil

Mix ingredients together.
Apply to affected areas.

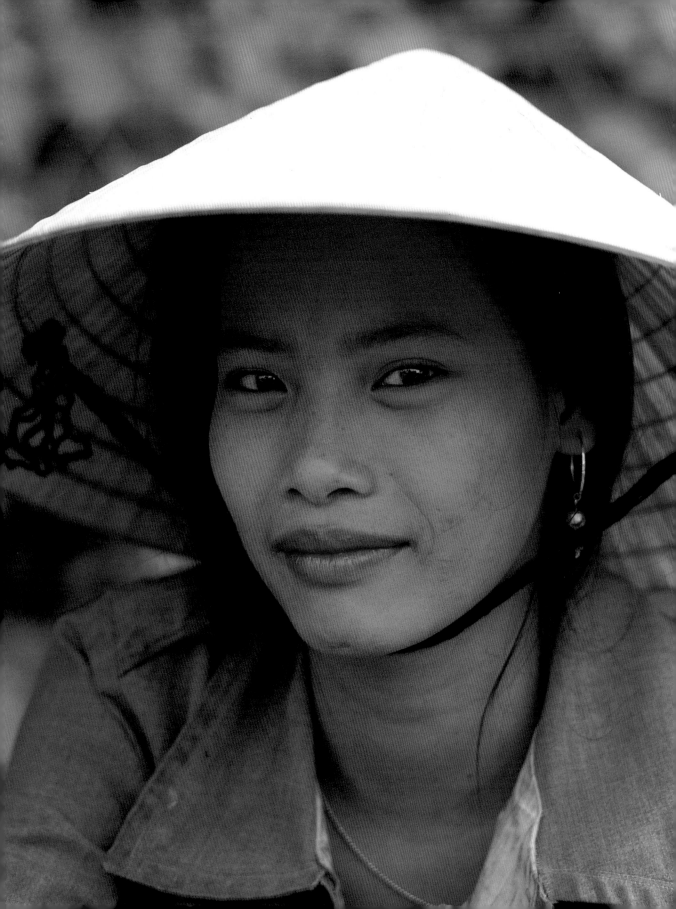

BEAUTY IS NATURE'S BRAG, AND MUST BE SHOWN
IN COURTS, AT FEASTS, AND HIGH SOLEMNITIES
WHERE MOST MAY WONDER AT THE WORKMANSHIP.
JOHN MILTON
English, 17th century
from "Comus"

Ylang-Ylang Mask

(for normal or oily skin)

Ylang-ylang is indigenous to the Maya Archi-
pelago. I noticed the women of Tahiti mixing
ylang-ylang with coconut oil, and using it as an
all-over body rub and in their hair.

1 teaspoon Wheatena brand cereal
1 teaspoon crushed oatmeal
1 teaspoon honey
1/2 cup plain yogurt
1 drop geranium oil
1 drop ylang-ylang oil

Warm the honey and combine it with the
yogurt, oatmeal, and Wheatena. Add the
essential oils and mix to make a thick paste.
Spread the paste onto your face and lie down
to relax. Leave the mask on for 10 to 20
minutes. Rinse off with tepid water.

Roman Conquest Mashed Fig Mask

Figs have been a popular fruit in Rome
since the conquest of Carthage.

1 small mashed banana
1 to 2 mashed figs

2 tablespoons oatmeal
2 tablespoons rosewater

Combine all the ingredients thoroughly
with a wooden spoon. Spread the paste onto
your face and lie down to relax. Leave the
mask on for 15 to 20 minutes.

A Rose Is a Rose Mask

Avocado and jojoba oil are used by women all
over Mexico to prevent premature aging, and to
keep their skin soft. This mask is excellent for
treating dry skin.

1/2 to 1 whole mashed avocado
1 to 2 tablespoons jojoba oil
1 to 2 capsules evening primrose oil
2 tablespoons heavy cream
1 drop rose oil
1 drop chamomile oil (optional)

Combine the avocado, jojoba and evening primrose oils, and the heavy cream to make a thick
paste. Add the rose and chamomile oils. Scoop
the paste up with your hands or a spatula, and
spread it onto your face. Leave the paste on
until it dries, then rinse off with tepid water.

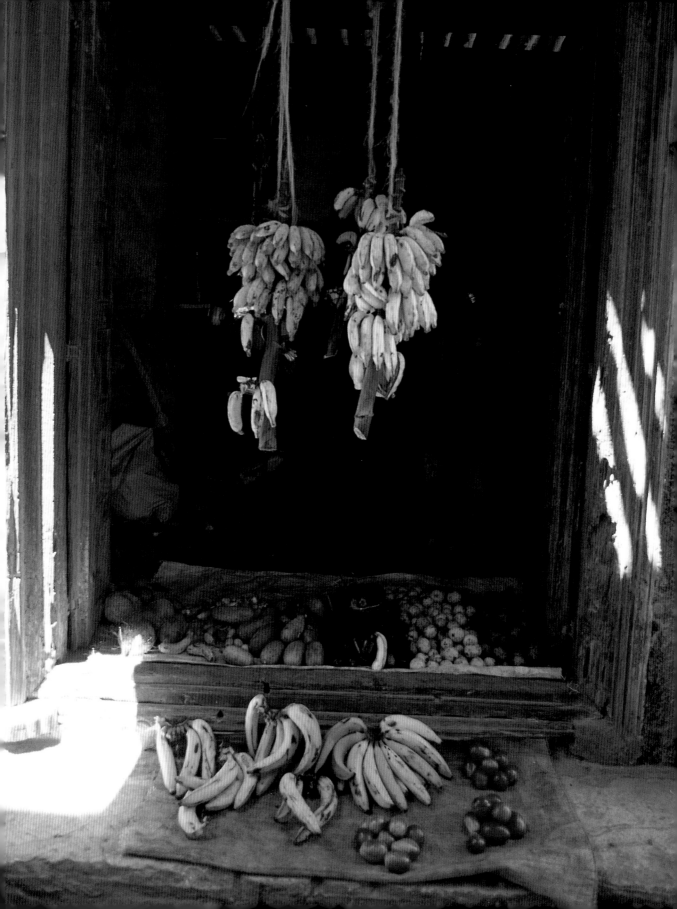

This is an easy way to whip up a soothing mask in a hurry. Start with a binding substance, like avocado, yogurt, or buttermilk (suitable for all skin types); or mud, clay, or oatmeal (nourishing to oily skin). Add to this base any of the following: banana, mayonnaise, bran, almonds, strawberries, tomatoes, essential oils, fruits, vegetables, vitamins E and A, or evening primrose oil. Watermelon, persimmon, and cucumber are the best match for skin pH, and cucumber is known to have antiwrinkle properties. You can mash any of these, add a bit of honey so they won't slip off your face, and apply them directly to the face, or combine them with a binding agent and apply the mixture.

Tsarina Mask

(for dry, mature skin)

This recipe is a favorite among Russian women. Wheat germ is rich in phosphorus and many vitamins such as vitamin E and is known to soothe, heal, and smooth wrinkles.

1 tablespoon wheat germ oil (available at grocery and health-food stores)
1 egg yolk, beaten
A few drops apple cider vinegar
2 capsules vitamin E (optional)

Whisk all the ingredients together and pat onto your face. Let dry for 10 to 15 minutes. Wash off with tepid water.

Masks for oily skin. If your face has excess oil, use any of the following base or binding substances, which have drying properties: buttermilk, plain yogurt, clay, or egg whites. Add a few drops of apple cider vinegar. Peel and mash any of the following fruits, and add to the binding substance: mango, grape, cranberry, apple, pineapple, grapefruit, lemon, or strawberry. The acids in these fruits help oily skin. Remember to test a small area first for any allergic reaction.

Masks for dry skin. For the base, use moisturizing substances, such as egg yolk, banana, honey, sour cream, or mayonnaise. Add a few drops of apple cider vinegar. People with dry skin will want to use fruits and vegetables with less acid, such as carrots (cooked until soft, then mashed), avocado, or canteloupe.

Papaya

Papaya contains an enzyme that can soften protein tissue. While traveling through the Caribbean, I marveled at how beautiful the women's complexions were, and I noticed they used papaya for cosmetic purposes. They used the ripe pulp as a soap, and used the juice to minimize wrinkles or freckles caused by the hot sun. Try massaging a bit of pulp into your skin, leaving it on for 5 minutes, then rinsing off.

Mexican Avocado Rub

The avocado has been a beauty secret of Latin American women since pre-Columbian times. The inside skin of the avocado is a wonderful exfoliant, adding vitamin E to your complexion. Remove the flesh of two avocados from their skins, and use in a salad. Rub the inside of the skin all over your face and neck. Leave on for a few minutes then wash off with tepid water. Or mash half of an avocado and apply directly to your face. Leave on for about 15 minutes then remove with lukewarm water.

Egyptian Clay Mask

(for oily skin)

Ancient Egyptians used clay masks and herbal masks as far back as 69–30 B.C., and masks are still very popular. Clays are completely natural and draw out toxins from deep within the skin. The term "fuller's earth" originated with fullers in cloth mills who used the clay to remove grease from fabric before it was sent to the market. You can find fuller's earth or any unbleached clay substance, such as kaolin, at health-food stores and pharmacies. If your skin is oily only in certain areas, you can just dot the areas that are blemished or oily.

Fuller's earth or kaolin clay (2 parts clay to 1 part water)
1 to 2 ripe tomatoes, papayas, or lemons

Combine clay mixture with the pulp of the fruit, adding water and mixing to create a smooth paste. Rub lightly into the skin, avoiding the eye area. Leave on for 10 to 15 minutes, or until dry. Wash off with warm or tepid water and then a cold splash.

Egyptian Clay Mask

(for dry skin)

Fuller's earth or kaolin clay (1 part clay to 1 part water)
1 teaspoon avocado or vegetable oil

Mix all the ingredients together in a ceramic bowl and apply to your face, avoiding the eye area. Leave on for 10 to 15 minutes, then rinse off. Note: Since clay can be drying, just dot the forehead, nose, and chin, if you like.

French Queen Beauty Mask

(for oily skin)

Marie Antoinette was famous for her beauty. Here is a treatment she might have enjoyed.

1/2 cup milk
1 to 2 teaspoons lemon juice
1 teaspoon brandy (optional)
A few drops apple cider vinegar

Combine all the ingredients in a saucepan and simmer over medium heat. Remove from the heat, let cool, and then apply to your face with a cotton pad. Leave on for about 15 minutes. Rinse off with cool water. Close pores with an astringent.

Egg, Almond, & Honey Mask

This delightful potion will leave your skin smooth and nourished.

1 egg yolk
1 teaspoon honey
1 teaspoon almond oil
1 teaspoon vitamin E oil
5 capsules evening primrose oil (optional)

Whisk all the ingredients together in a mixing bowl. Prick the oil capsules with a pin and add the oil to the mixture. Slather onto your face and leave on for 10 to 15 minutes.
Rinse off with tepid water.

Scottish Oatmeal Mask

Oatmeal comforts and nourishes the skin. It is naturally gentle and mild—perfect for people with sensitive skin. Scottish, Irish, and Indian women have been using oatmeal for centuries to soften and heal their complexions. For oily skin, omit the oil and add 1 tablespoon lemon juice and half of a mashed apple. If your skin is dry, add half of a mashed banana and 1 tablespoon honey.

1/2 cup cooked, cooled oatmeal
1 whole egg
1 tablespoon almond oil

Combine all the ingredients and apply to your face. Leave on for 10 minutes, then rinse off with warm water.

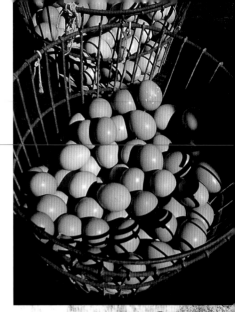

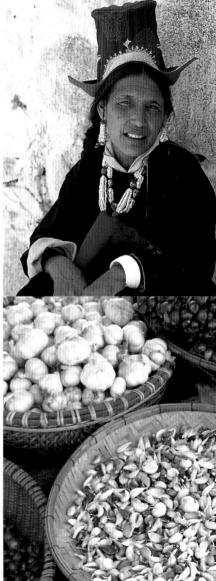

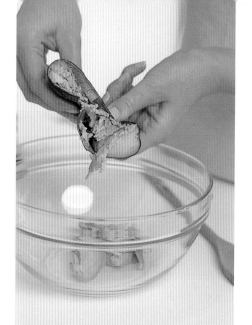

Aztec Crushed Avocado Mask
(for dry skin)

Women in South America
and Mexico have been using
avocado for their hair and
skin for thousands of years
as a protective barrier from the
sun. It contains vitamin E and
is extremely nourishing.

1 average sized avocado, mashed
1 ripe banana, mashed
1 teaspoon honey

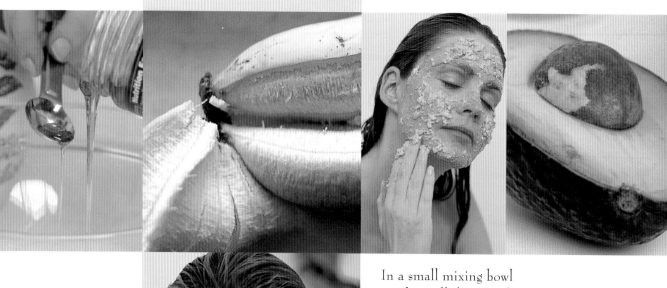

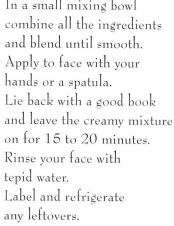

In a small mixing bowl
combine all the ingredients
and blend until smooth.
Apply to face with your
hands or a spatula.
Lie back with a good book
and leave the creamy mixture
on for 15 to 20 minutes.
Rinse your face with
tepid water.
Label and refrigerate
any leftovers.

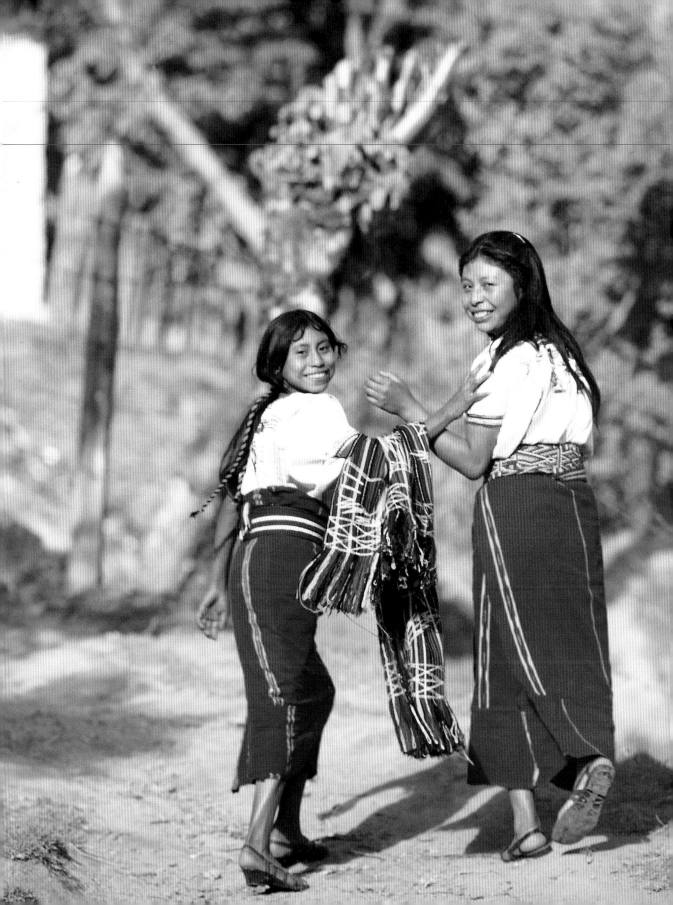

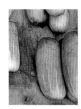
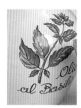
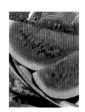

Summer Splash Cucumber Mask

This is a perfect recipe for those hot, sticky summer days. Cucumbers are a natural astringent, and this mask will tighten your skin. It's like having a mini face-lift. Wrinkles seem to soften and diminish after using this mask.

1 small cucumber
1 to 2 tablespoons skim milk
1 teaspoon honey
A few drops apple cider vinegar
Several teaspoons crushed ice

Chop the cucumber into small pieces and put in a blender. Add the milk, honey, vinegar, and ice. Blend until smooth and creamy. Do not let the mixture get runny. Spread all over your face and neck. Sit down and relax with soft music. You can also put cucumber slices on your eyes. Leave on for about 15 minutes, then rinse off with cold water or a cool shower.

Pueblo Fresh Watermelon Mask

Among the Pueblo Indians, watermelon was so highly regarded that these juicy fruits were often given as gifts during ceremonies and special occasions. The Pueblos believed that watermelon juice renews the blood. I always seem to have watermelon around in the summer because it's such a great snack or dessert.

1 cup watermelon

Mash the fruit in a small mixing bowl until smooth. Apply liberally to the face and cover with a moist washcloth, or add a binding substance (yogurt for oily skin or banana for dry skin) to keep the mask from sliding off.

Yogurt Lemon Mask

When yogurt is used regularly, it nourishes and smoothes the texture of the skin. It is loaded with calcium.

1/2 cup plain yogurt
5 drops lemon juice

Combine the ingredients, apply to your face, and leave the mask on while you relax in the bath. The mask will tighten. When finished with your bath remove the mask with splashes of cool water.

Mediterranean Olive Oil Treatment

In the Mediterranean, olive oil is the cooking oil of choice. My Italian grandmother always used olive oil in her recipes. It is wonderful for dry, wrinkled, or parched skin. Warm a few tablespoons of olive oil. Smooth it all over your face, neck, and chest. Allow the oil to penetrate your skin as you relax in the bath. This wonderful oil helps eliminate wrinkles and rejuvenates the complexion. Rinse off at the end of your bath.

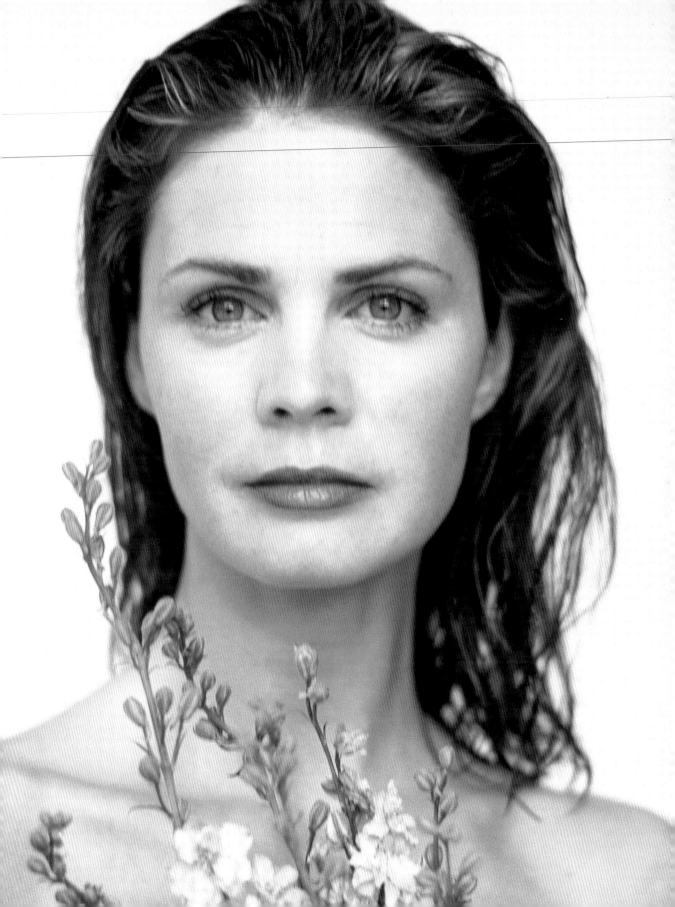

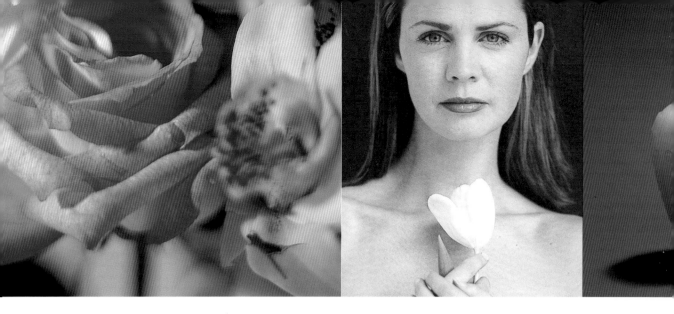

HOW TO GIVE YOURSELF A FACIAL

1   Set the stage with soft music and an aromatherapy candle.

2   Cleanse your face thoroughly before you begin. Make sure all makeup is removed.

3   Steam your face to eliminate toxins (if you have sensitive skin or broken capillaries, use a warm compress instead).

4   Apply a face mask to deep-clean the skin (use any of the recipes below, depending on skin type).

5   Sit back and relax with a good book or soft music for 15 to 20 minutes.

6   Rinse your face thoroughly with tepid water.

7   Tone your face with an herbal toner or an herbal astringent.

8   Moisturize. Massage your face with a cream, light oil, or lotion. Make sure you also moisturize the'neck.

Claudine's Quick Facial

My friend Claudine is a great athlete, a fitness trainer, and a gorgeous African American model. She gave me this quick beauty treatment, which she says helps her prevent breakouts. She also recommends getting lots of exercise, as sweating helps to remove toxins from your body.

1   Steam your face over a bowl of freshly boiled water with a towel over your head.

2   Apply a mask of either egg whites or mashed banana with honey.

3   Cover your eyes with cucumber to take away any puffiness.

4   Rinse your face when the mask dries.

5   Tone with witch hazel.

6   Conclude with lots of moisturizer.

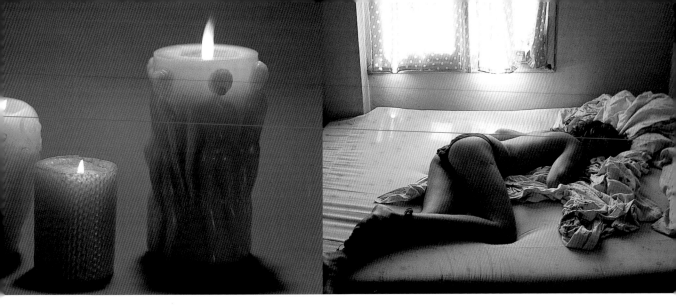

Josephine de Beaubarais Facial

(for normal or oily skin)

Napoleon's wife was not a conventional beauty, but men found her captivating nonetheless. She created a scandal with her extravagant beauty regimes and enormous clothing bills. Brought up in Martinique in the West Indies, she brought many New World beauty secrets with her to the Imperial court in Paris.

1 egg white, beaten
1 tablespoon honey
A few drops apple cider vinegar

Beat the egg white until frothy, then add the remaining ingredients. Spread over your face and leave on for a few minutes. Rinse off with tepid water.

Josephine de Beaubarais Facial

(for dry skin)

1 egg yolk, beaten
1 tablespoon honey
1 tablespoon almond oil
A few drops apple cider vinegar

Beat the egg white until smooth, then add the remaining ingredients. Spread over your face and leave on for a few minutes. Rinse off with tepid water.

Aphrodite's Facial

(for oily skin)

Brewers' yeast was used by the early Greeks and Romans for medicinal purposes; it has deep-cleaning action and is rich in vitamins, minerals, and proteins.

1 tablespoon brewers' yeast
1 to 2 tablespoons warm water or warm milk
1 tablespoon almond oil or sesame oil
1 egg yolk

First spread a thin coat of almond oil on your face. Then combine all the ingredients and blend to make a thick paste. Spread a light coat over the almond oil and leave on for 10 to 15 minutes. Use a soft, clean washcloth or splash with tepid water to remove.

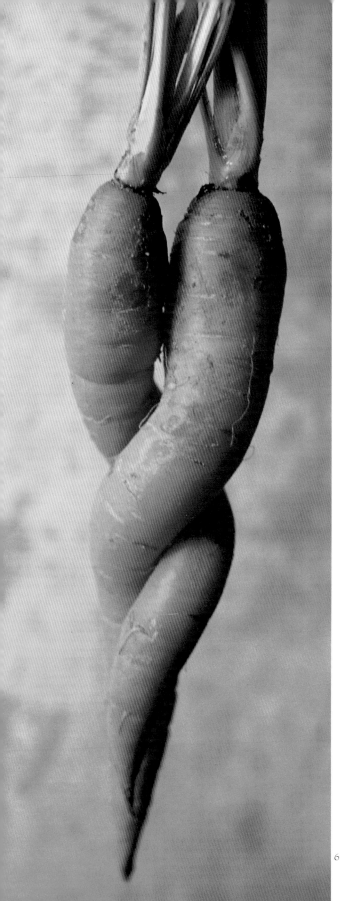

What's up, Doc?
Cooked Carrot Facial

(for dry skin)

Carrots are rich in vitamin A. They make wonderful facials and are vital for healthy skin. A friend of mine brought this recipe back from a visit to Hungary. You can use turnips in place of the carrots.

1 to 2 cooked mashed carrots
1/2 teaspoon wheat germ oil
1 to 2 teaspoons honey
2 drops geranium oil (optional)

Combine all the ingredients in a bowl. Slather the mixture onto your face. Leave on for 20 minutes, then rinse off.

Mini-Quickie Facials

If you're in a hurry and don't have time for a complete facial, put on a simple one- or two-ingredient mask. Avocado, yogurt, and egg masks are easy to prepare and are effective after a short time on your face. Blend, apply, and leave the mask on your face for 5 or 10 minutes. Jump in the shower or wash your face with cool water.

Cucumber juice
Nature's perfect "liquid rejuvenator."
Keeps the skin youthful and radiant.
A great skin toner and the ultimate
sunburn and wrinkle treatment.

Apple juice
High in silicon and malic acid. Silicon is
great for skin, hair, and nails. The malic acid
in apple juice is said to flush out cellulite.

Orange and grapefruit juices
Necessary for skin's collagen. High in
vitamin C, calcium, and phosphorus.

Mango juice
While traveling in India I noticed that mango
juice was frequently used as a delicious drink
to relieve dehydration.

Asparagus juice
Helps clear up blemishes by
neutralizing excess acid.

Watermelon juice
Flushes acid from the system
and the blood.

Berry juice
Raspberries, blueberries, and
strawberries should be a routine part
of a woman's diet since they are rich in
vitamin C and iron.

Carrot juice
Carrot juice contains all the vitamins
and minerals for beautiful skin and hair.
Carrot juice helps clear blemishes
and heal dry skin.

Quick Beauty Secrets

- Aloe vera is very healing when applied topically. Use the gel straight from the plant or use the all-natural bottled gel, but make sure it doesn't include synthetics.

- Half a cup of apple cider vinegar mixed with 1/2 cup water makes a wonderful face rinse.

- Honey is very healing. Dab a small amount directly on a blemish to help it disappear. Try unfiltered honey, which retains all the important nutrients and enzymes.

- Aveeno (colloidal oatmeal) found at the pharmacy is wonderful for dry, itchy skin.

- Drinking 8 to 10 glasses of water a day will hydrate your skin and make it beautiful.

- The lactic acid found in milk treatments keeps skin youthful and beautiful.

- Tea tree oil is great for blemishes; just dab a little on problem spots.

- Always wear sunscreen. Most wrinkles are caused by sun damage.

SLEEP

Everyone experiences sleepless nights due to anxiety, worrying about
the day's events, too much caffeine, eating too much or too late in the day.
A good night's sleep produces a feeling of well-being. You feel energized, ready
to conquer the day, and your eyes are radiant. Natural therapies are best; avoid
commercial sleeping pills. Natural therapies are also nonaddictive.

- Take a warm bath an hour or two before bedtime for about 20 to 30 minutes
  (see bathing recipes). It will raise your body temperature and improve sleep.
- Take a cold 1-to-3 minute foot bath with water up to your calves.
- Kneel or sit in cold water so that the thighs are covered, or sit in cold water that
  reaches just to your stomach for 3 to 5 minutes. It regulates circulation and helps
  you fall asleep.
- Try to avoid all caffeine after two in the afternoon. Caffeine can cause
  insomnia and can wake you up in the middle of the night.
- Drink a small glass of mineral water before bed.
- Avoid heavy meals in the evening and try not to eat right before bed.
- Avoid salty and sugary foods before your bedtime.
- If you live near an airport or busy street try a white-noise machine, a fan, or earplugs.
- Try drinking a cup of chamomile or peppermint tea before bed. Chamomile tea
  is also good for menstrual cramps.
- Drink a glass of warm skim milk with 1 tablespoon of honey.
- Take two tablets of calcium with magnesium.
- Celery, bananas, brown rice, lemon water with honey, warm milk with honey, and
  wheat germ are good sleepy-time snacks about an hour before you go to bed.
- Do not exercise right before bed. Exercise in the morning or at least 5 hours
  before bedtime.
- Gaze at a lighted candle for a few minutes before you go to bed.
- Take 10 deep breaths; wait 5 minutes, then take 10 more.
- Try autosuggestion: lie on your back and think of each body part as heavy
  and relaxed. Start with the feet and slowly move up to your head.

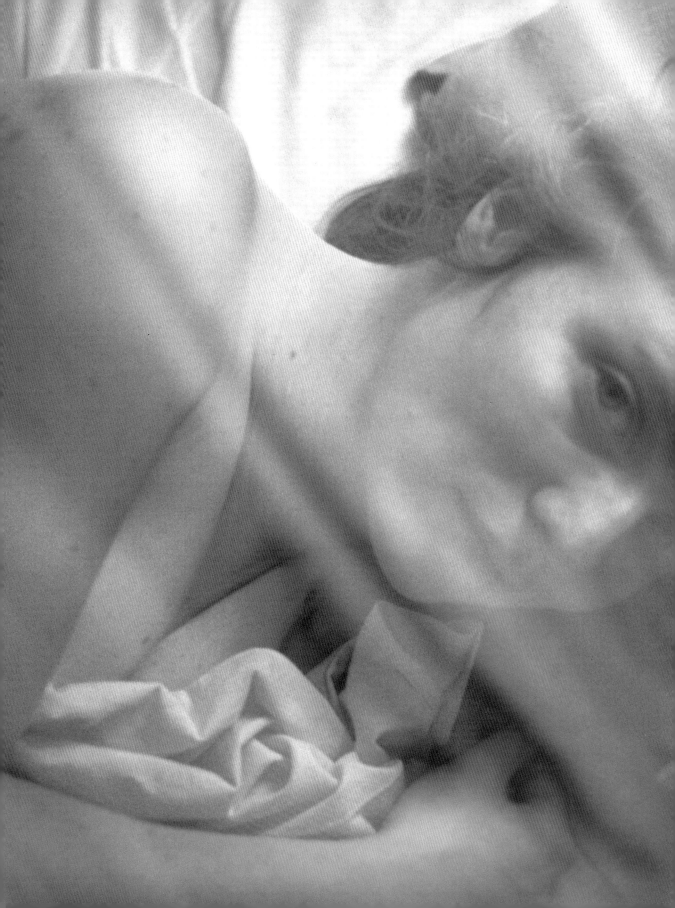

I SING THE BODY ELECTRIC . . .
WAS IT DOUBTED THAT THOSE WHO CORRUPT THEIR BODIES CONCEAL THEMSELVES? . . .
AND IF THE BODY DOES NOT DO FULLY AS MUCH AS THE SOUL?
AND IF THE BODY WERE NOT THE SOUL, WHAT IS THE SOUL?

WALT WHITMAN
American, 19th century
from "Children of Adam"

THE BODY

Indigenous peoples, tribes who live on the lands of their forefathers, believe the human body is a temple of the spirit. The Judeo-Christian tradition maintains in the Book of Genesis that God created man in his own image. Yet, although we moderns have been known to worship bodies, rarely are they our own.

Stress, environmental pollutants, bad diets, fad diets, too much or too little exercise—these are some of the reasons a woman's body can get knocked out of balance, or corrupt, as Whitman might say. Whatever shape the body is in, it

deserves respect and a little pampering. This chapter is full of simple ways to soothe and coax your body back into balance, through bathing, thalassotherapy (sea water treatment), and massage. It also explains how to enhance a bath or massage with soothing or stimulating aromatherapy oils you create yourself. These are all simple things that can easily fit into even the busiest schedule.

The ultimate goal is not to achieve a predetermined ideal of bodily perfection. Too often, women have been made to feel ashamed of

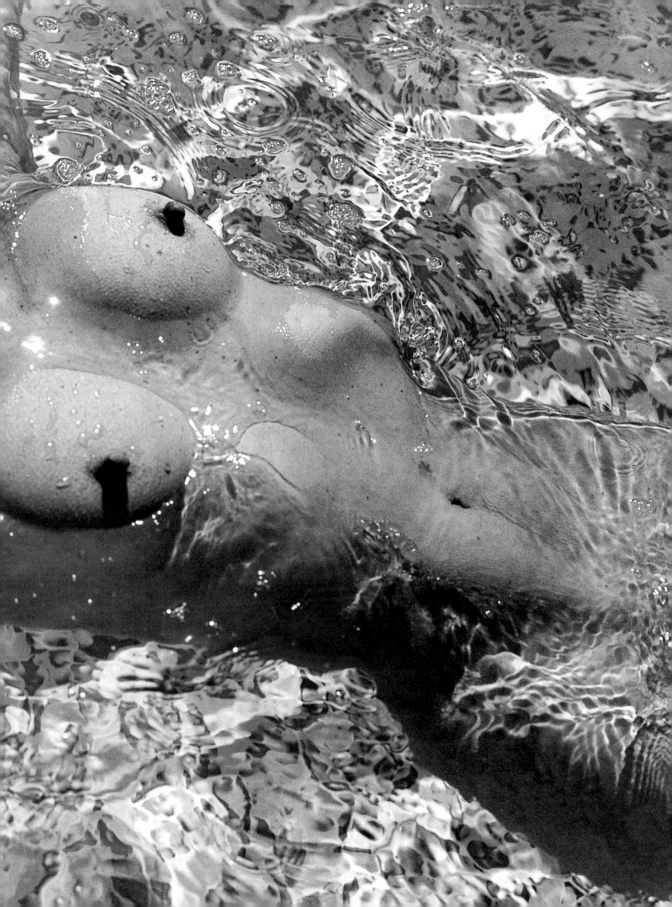

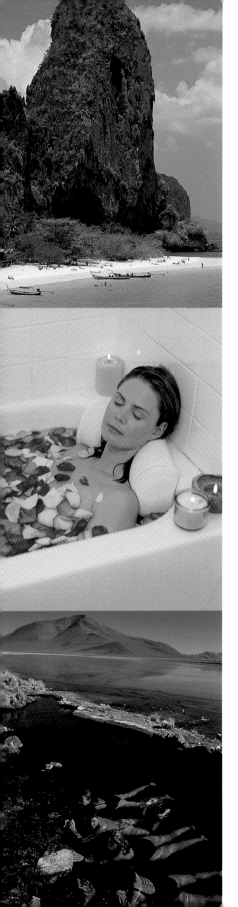

bodies that don't conform to the current notion of feminine beauty, be it the blowzy zaftig figure of the seventeenth century, or the waiflike thinness of the late twentieth century.

This chapter will assist you in achieving the best for the natural shape of your body, whether it's deliciously curvaceous or charmingly petite. Working with your natural body design, treating yourself to an invigorating bath or a soothing massage—here you'll find the tools to give your body lift and life. When you have a true sense of personal well-being, a sense of pride in the beauty and sensuality you possess should follow as a matter of course.

And here's a bonus: bodily equilibrium yields emotional benefits. Practitioners of modern medicine and psychology congratulate themselves on the "discovery" of the body-mind connection, a concept often associated with Eastern religious and medical practices. But cultures throughout the world have long believed that the mind and body are not different, discrete units. Ironically, leading-edge Western researchers are coming to much the same conclusion. They theorize that the mind is not limited to a gray, crenulated organ in the skull; rather, the mind encompasses the body's entire network of signals and impulses, sensing, feeling, and reacting.

This lends credence to the idea that body and mind are essentially inseparable, and that well-being depends on a holistic approach to body care. Body-care products and processes that ease and improve the mind as well as the body are much more effective than those that tend only to the physical needs of the body.

INDIANS AND ANIMALS KNOW BETTER HOW TO LIVE THAN WHITE MAN;
NOBODY CAN BE IN GOOD HEALTH IF HE DOES NOT HAVE ALL THE
TIME, FRESH AIR, SUNSHINE, AND GOOD WATER.

FLYING HAWK
Oglala Sioux, 19th to 20th century

BATHING

Descended as we are, through evolutionary millennia, from sea-borne, single-celled creatures, life without water is inconceivable, impossible. The absolute necessity of water has been acknowledged by all civilizations since recorded history. Early on, and throughout the world, water took on a mystical weight and significance beyond its more prosaic uses.

Bathing has always had many religious connotations, notably in the Christian rite of baptism, performed to wash away the stain of original sin. Rosewater has been used since the Middle Ages to purify mosques. Celtic peoples worshipped water. They believed the gods resided in the waters, and certain hot springs (those at present-day Bath, England, for instance) were sacred to Sulis, the sun deity.

Bathing has also been a social activity around the world; the Romans were especially famous for it. Their immense and impressive Baths of Caracalla served the imperial and general populace with hot, warm, and cold pools, as well as steam and exercise rooms, libraries, and lecture halls.

Medicinal powers have long been attributed to thermal and mineral baths. In the fifth century B.C., Hippocrates extolled water's beneficial effects on the body. In the nineteenth century, people took the waters, drinking and soaking away their ills. Kaisers and kings decamped for the season to fashionable spas like Eugénie-les-Bains, Baden-Baden, and Karlovy Vary, pursued by a retinue of poets, musicians, and mistresses. Modern European physicians still prescribe hydrotherapy cures.

For many women, however, bathing has become a pedestrian exercise in basic hygiene. The daily shower is the ablutionary equivalent of fast food—brusque, bland, and ultimately unsatisfying as a regular diet. A boring bath is a manifestation of the too-busy life. Fortunately, it's simple to transform bathing into a rejuvenating sensual pleasure—as it has been since the days of Cleopatra.

Bathing can be relaxing or energizing, depending on things like water temperature, and bath oils and salts. Different herbs and oils can create a bath that's soothing. A bath softens the skin and replaces moisture. Water opens the pores, drawing out sweat and toxins, and restores to skin a clearer, smoother, more glowing finish.

SEMI-BATH

In the nineteenth century, Father Kneipp, a Swiss expert on hydrotherapy and herbs, suggested a three- to five-minute cold bath. He encouraged his clients to kneel so the water covered the thighs, or to sit so the water reached the stomach. The semi-bath is not only a sleep aid; it also can act as a morning-after antidote to a poor night's rest.

Water Temperature

The temperature of the bath or shower is largely a matter of taste; however, it's important to understand the effects of different water temperatures. Although many people love a scalding hot bath or shower, temperatures over 100 degrees sap skin of its moisture. Water temperature close to body temperature, between 90 and 100 degrees, is optimal. If you're addicted to heat, a steam bath (in which the water never touches the skin) is preferable.

Warm water temperatures are best for relaxing. The heat also helps release the fragrance, and maximize the healing and cleansing effects, of salts and oils.

Cold water temperatures are stimulating. A cool bath or shower enhances circulation, waking up the entire system. When used regularly, cold bathing can help increase resistance to colds and infections and improve digestion.

TOOLS OF THE TRADE

The most important piece of equipment is, of course, the tub or shower. Optimally, a tub allows you to stretch out, so that the body can be totally submerged up to the neck. Always use a non-slip mat. Japanese homes often have an upright tub, much like a box, in which the bather sits on a low stool. Shower design is getting ever more exotic, with vertical jets up the sides of the shower stall to reach all parts of the body.

Keep in mind, however, that water is a precious resource (requiring additional resources for purification and heating), and should be used sparingly. Tubs use up much more water than showers—so try bathing with a partner. Earth-friendly showerheads, which use less water, are also available. They give off a finer, mist-like spray, which is pleasant, as well as easier on dry skin than a heavy, pounding flow.

Bath or shower, both work better with a few extras: a bath pillow to rest your head; an aromatherapy candle; some large, absorbent cotton towels. A natural sponge is far superior to anything man-made. Natural sponges can be incredibly soft or invigoratingly rough, and very absorbent. The best are known as Turkey sponges and have many tiny holes; the smaller the holes, the better (and probably more costly) the sponge. A loofah is made from a member of the gourd family. Loofahs give a stimulating massage and their fine network of filaments sloughs off dead surface skin cells. A regular loofah rub can prevent ingrown hairs—great for areas that are shaved or waxed. A pumice stone is useful for smoothing the roughest spots like heels, elbows, and knees.

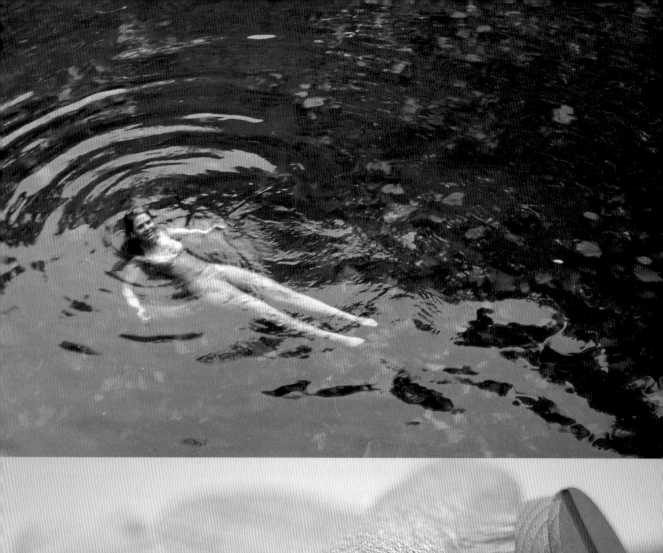

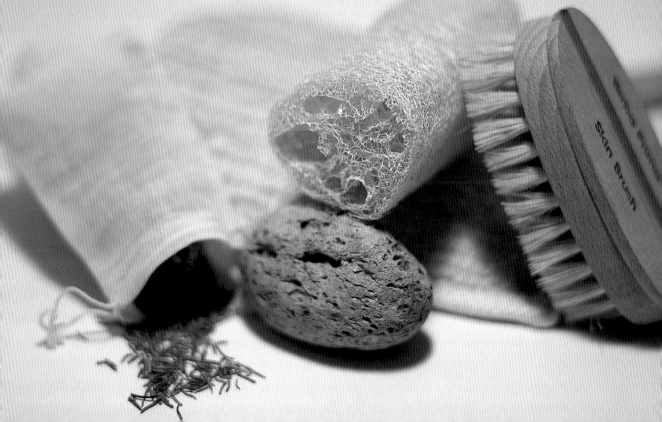

Flemish Fields Soothing Oatmeal Bath

Oats have traditionally been an important crop in northern Europe and an integral part of the cereal production system since the Middle Ages. In their triennial system of crop rotation, lowland farmers divided up arable land into three fields, one containing oats, one wheat, one fallow. While the peasants needed every grain for sustenance, among the burghers of Bruges or Antwerp (Europe's most important fragrance and spice market in the sixteenth century), the ladies might have afforded themselves the luxury of an oatmeal bath enhanced with a hint of vanilla—a whiff of tropical America.

1 cup oatmeal (or almond- or cornmeal)
1 1/2 cup warm milk or warm water
1 tablespoon honey
1 tablespoon vanilla extract

Combine all ingredients in a blender or food processor until smooth. Smaller particles make for a richer bath and prevent a clogged drain. Pour under running water into the bath. Soak in the bath for 20 to 30 minutes, then finish off with a cold sponging or shower.

Queen of the Nile Milk Bath

Thus did Shakespeare imagine Cleopatra's fateful sail up the Nile to her first meeting with Mark Antony. Cleopatra had a vast array of potions and perfumes at hand to enhance her allure.

The ancient Egyptians were, in fact, masters of the cosmetic arts. Many artifacts discovered in royal tombs are vessels filled with rare spices and precious oils, and portraits show feminine faces enhanced by beauty products. Cleopatra was famous for milk and almond baths. For centuries, milk has been used to smooth dry, lifeless skin; and almonds contain vitamins, minerals, and proteins that further nourish the complexion. Chamomile has softening properties.

4 cups whole milk or the equivalent of powdered milk
15 tablespoons almond meal
3 tablespoons honey
1/2 cup chamomile infusion (optional)

Whisk together all of the ingredients for several minutes, until thoroughly blended. Add a cup of the mixture to warm bath water. Store the remainder in a covered, labeled jar for use throughout the week.

BATHING SECRETS

1 Try adding a cup of apple cider vinegar to your bath. It works wonders for dry, itchy, flaky skin.

2 I like to place two to three chamomile or peppermint tea bags in my bath.

3 If you have aches and pains, try placing a few crushed aspirin into your bath water.

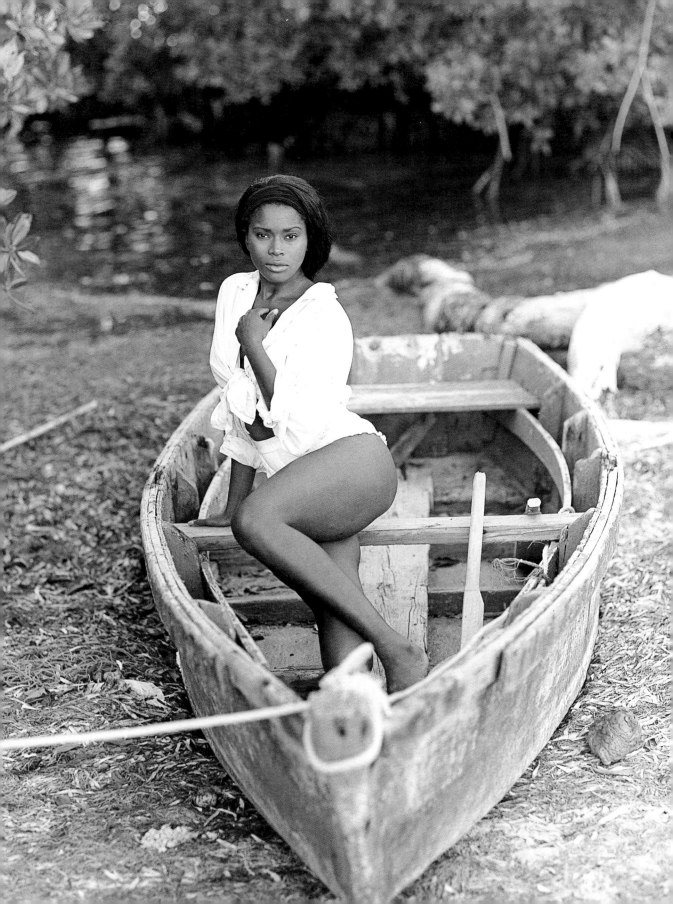

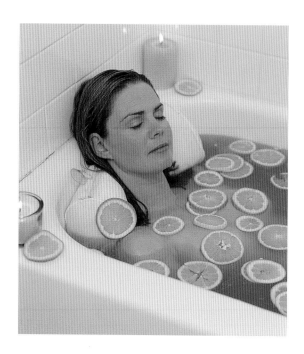

Orange Juice Bath

The vitamin C in this bath will revitalize and rejuvenate your skin. Plus, it will cool you off.

2 to 3 ripe oranges
2 to 3 fresh lemons (optional)

Fill the tub with warm water. Cut the oranges and lemons in half and squeeze the juice into the tub. Then, if you want, cut the orange and lemon halves into slices and place them in the warm water. Lie back with a good book and soak for 15 to 20 minutes. Step out and pat the skin lightly with a towel. The vitamin C will absorb into the skin, leaving you feeling refreshed.

Rose Petal Bath

1 to 3 cups rose petals
1 tablespoon lavender flowers (optional)
1 to 2 drops rose oil

The rose has always been a symbol of love. This bath is the ultimate luxury and perfect for a romantic evening. Fill the tub with warm water, dropping in the rose oil. Sprinkle the rose petals on top of the water. Enjoy the petals floating around you as you soak.

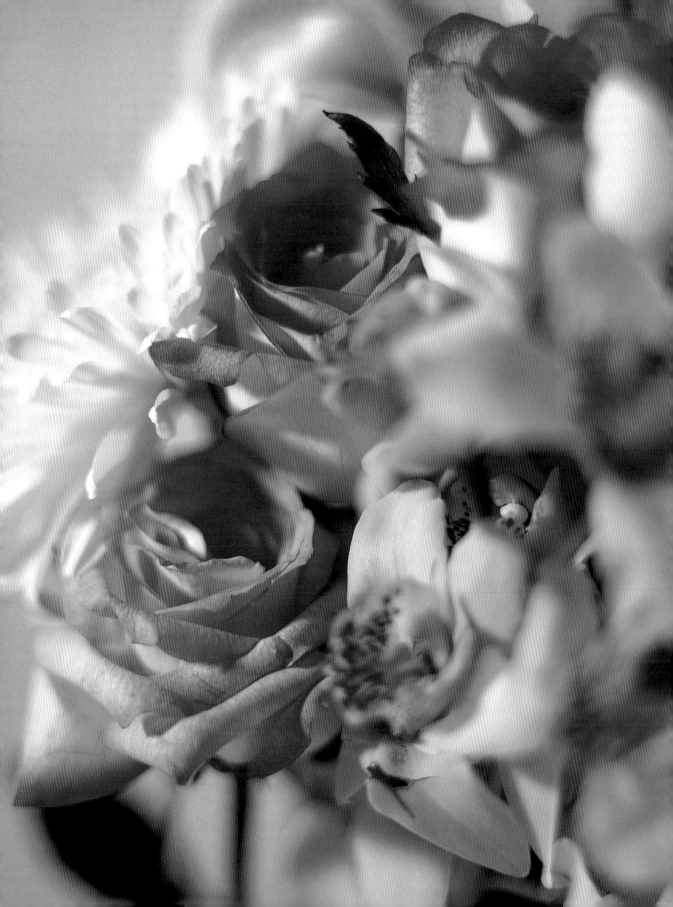

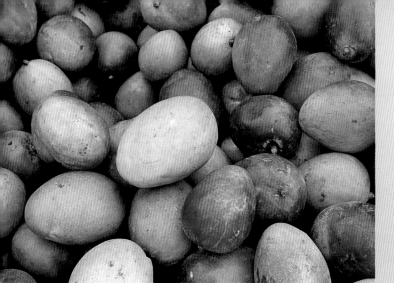
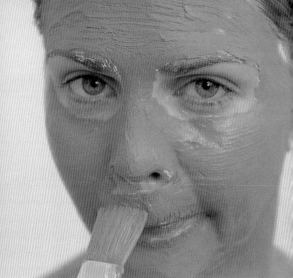

Tropical Paradise Body Scrub

The mango tree, which can grow as tall as forty or fifty feet, probably originated in southeast Asia, where its lush, evergreen foliage is a welcome source of shade. Buddha was given a mango grove to help him keep cool during meditation.

Many Caribbean women use fresh fruits and vegetables to keep their complexions clear and fresh in the hot tropical sun. While traveling in the Islands I noticed women using papaya or mango to slough off dead skin cells. This scrub is redolent with fresh fruit and has a touch of vinegar for cleansing. The scent of the fruits will whisk you off to a steamy, sensual equatorial island.

1 small ripe mango
1 small ripe papaya (optional)
1/4 cup water
3 to 4 tablespoons oatmeal (or cornmeal)
1 teaspoon cider vinegar
1 tablespoon honey

Remove the peel and pit from the mango. Either mash the fruit in a bowl or mix it in your blender or food processor. Add the oats, vinegar, water, and honey, and whisk or blend until the mixture forms a paste. Use in the shower as an all-over body treatment and gentle exfoliant. Rinse with tepid, then cool water. Pat skin dry.

For a quick treatment, you can also rub the inside of a papaya or mango skin over your body and face. The small fibers of the inner skin will leave your skin feeling soft. Leave the residue on for 5 to 10 minutes and then rinse off.

Kyoto Sea Kelp Body Mask

Seaweed is part of the Japanese and Pacific Islanders' diet, and Japanese skin-care specialists use marine plants for their healing properties. This nourishing all-over body mask removes toxins and renews the skin.

1/2 cup powdered French clay
1 to 2 teaspoons almond oil
A few drops vitamin E oil
1/4 cup warm water
One pinch sea salt
1 teaspoon powdered kelp

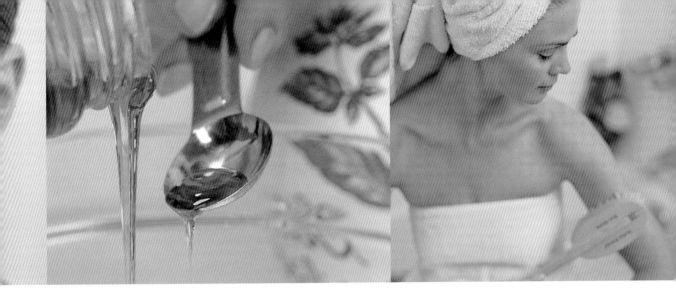

Mix the clay and water first, then add the oils to make a smooth paste. Spread the mask all over the face and body, using your hands or a paintbrush. Leave on for 10 to 15 minutes then rinse off with cool water.

Do not allow it to dry completely, as masks can be very dehydrating. If you have dry skin, add a mashed avocado. Avoid clay masks if you have very sensitive skin.

Persian Honey and Yogurt Body Treatment

This wonderful body treatment, rich in vitamins, calcium, and protein, would please any pasha. Honey has been used in body and facial treatments around the world for centuries. I noticed while traveling that Balinese women use sweet honey as a body mask. Honey contains potassium; it softens and heals the skin, while fighting bacteria. Wheat germ is a good exfoliant.

2 cups plain yogurt
1 to 2 tablespoons wheat germ
1 teaspoon honey
2 egg whites (for oily skin) or
1 mashed banana (for dry skin)

Combine the ingredients and apply all over the body and hair. Leave on for 5 minutes then rinse off. Conditions, cleanses, and moisturizes.

DRY SKIN BRUSHING

Dry skin brushing is said to remove toxins from the body and enhance the immune system. Brushing your skin regularly can help decrease cellulite by improving blood circulation and muscle tone. Your body will feel invigorated and your skin will look younger and better. Use a dry brush with natural bristles (available at health food stores) and a long handle so you can reach your back. Do not wet the brush. Start at the feet and brush in circular movements gradually moving up. Massage the entire body—the thighs, buttocks, abdomen, back, hands, and arms—for about 5 minutes or until your skin is pink. Do not brush irritated skin or your face. Then jump in your shower or bath. Clean the brush with warm water and soap and let it dry naturally.

Oh let me flow into the ocean,
Let me get back to the sea.
Let me be stormy and let me be calm,
Let the tide in, and set me free.

Pete Townshend
English, 20th century
from "Drowned"

Thalassotherapy

Thalassa is the Greek word for sea. The nineteenth-century French physician Dr. Stephan Bonnardiere coined the term thalassotherapy, advising his patients to get plenty of exposure to sea air and salt water to maintain good health, or to take an ocean voyage to cure illness. Thalassotherapy became fashionable, quite simply, because it works. In the nineteenth century, the coasts of the Atlantic, Mediterranean, and Black Sea were lined with spas offering all kinds of treatments based on seawater and marine vegetation.

Modern scientists speculate that visiting the seaside can be healthful because the churning water releases positive ions that are beneficial to the body's metabolic processes (Hampton, 62–3). Our skin resembles the protective outer layers of plants in structure and function; elements found in salt water and marine plants are similar to the chemical makeup of human plasma. The oceans' minerals are full of nutrients good for skin, hair, and internal organs. Sea plants contain such vital elements as potassium, beta-carotene, and iodine, in concentrations greater than those found in land-grown plants.

Seawater is often used to treat the aches and pains of skeleto-muscular conditions like arthritis. It also promotes healing of certain wounds and rashes. Spas use thalassotherapy for everything from improving the complexion to reducing cellulite, incorporating salt water and seaweed, kelp and other marine herbs into baths, jet sprays, and body wraps. The simplest way to enjoy a little thalassotherapy at home is to incorporate it occasionally into your bath routine.

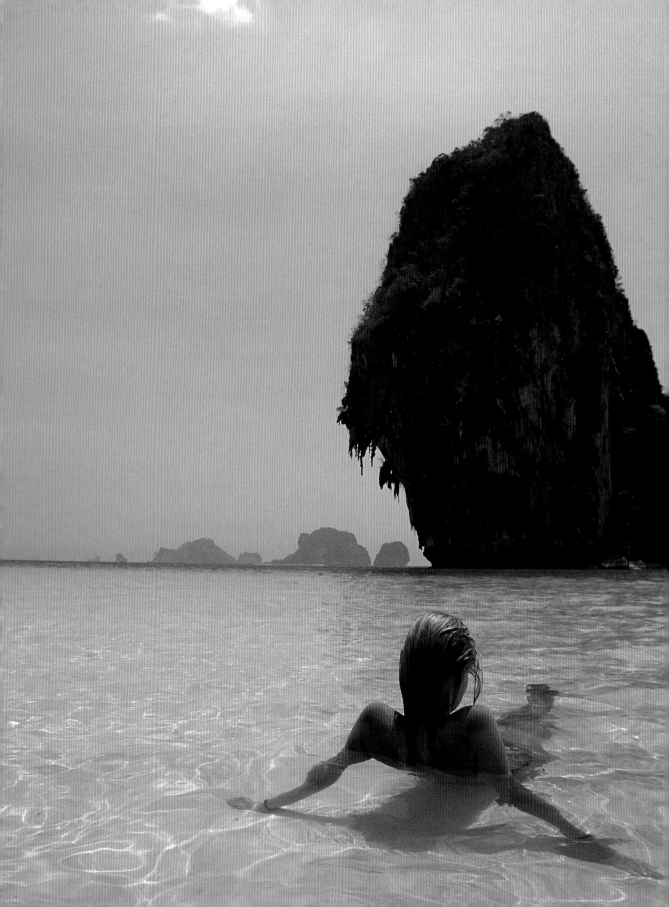

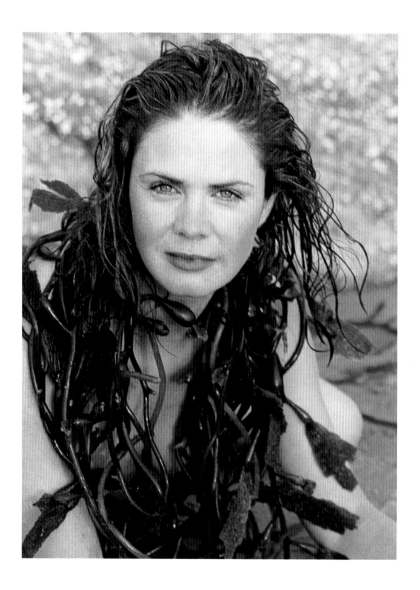

Poseidon Seaweed Bath

Seaweed is wonderful therapy for dry skin, containing revitalizing elements like iodine and protein. While working as a model in Japan, I met several Japanese women who told me that eating seaweed and kelp contributed to their beautiful skin. They believe that what they eat is very important for maintaining outer beauty. They also use seaweed in their bath treatments.

You can create a mini-ocean at home with dehydrated seaweed, available at many health-food stores; or if there's a beach nearby, gather an armful of seaweed, rinse thoroughly, and add to your bath. Try collecting different kinds, testing them one at a time and finding a combination that you prefer. Draw a warm bath and add the seaweed. After soaking, rinse off any oil or residue from your body. Discard seaweed after use.

I AM ONE OF NATURE'S CHILDREN
AND WHENEVER I SEE HER, PLEASURE ROLL IN MY BREAST,
AND SWELL AND BURST LIKE WAVES ON THE SHORE OF THE OCEAN,
IN PRAYER AND PRAISE TO HIM WHO HAS PLACED ME IN HER HAND.

GEORGE COPWAY

Native American, 20th century

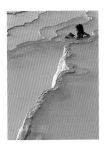

Big Sur Sea Salt Scrub

This scrub and skin toner is a favorite at West Coast spas that specialize in natural and organic therapy. It's perfect for soaking in a hot tub high above the pounding Pacific surf. The salt has a wonderful tingling effect as it soothes and draws toxins out of your skin. I love to massage myself with this paste to give my skin an extra glow and all-over energy.

2 cups coarse sea salt (preferably Kosher or Diamond brand)
1/2 cup almond oil
1 tablespoon sesame oil (optional)

Combine all the ingredients into a paste. This recipe can be messy, so you might want to apply it in the tub. Dip a natural sponge into the paste and rub all over the body (avoiding the face and groin) with a circular motion. Leave the paste on your skin, and relax for 5 to 10 minutes, enjoying the tingle. Rinse with warm water followed by a cold splash. This recipe does not require refrigeration so you can keep a batch in a pretty jar in your bathroom.

Israeli Dead Sea Mineral Bath

My Israeli friend Hanna told me that women in Israel use mud and salt from the Dead Sea for many beauty treatments. She believes that the Dead Sea contains all the minerals the skin needs to look beautiful. She recently brought back some Dead Sea salts as a gift for my bath, and it was heavenly.

This is a mixture for relaxing. You can use it as is or add aromatherapy oils to enhance its soothing, restorative powers.

1/2 cup Dead Sea Salts (available in specialty health and beauty stores)
1/2 cup Epsom salts (optional)
1/2 cup baking soda
2 to 3 drops chamomile oil (optional)
2 to 3 drops lavender oil (optional)

Combine the ingredients and add to a bath. Add chamomile oil or lavender oil for an even more relaxing soak.

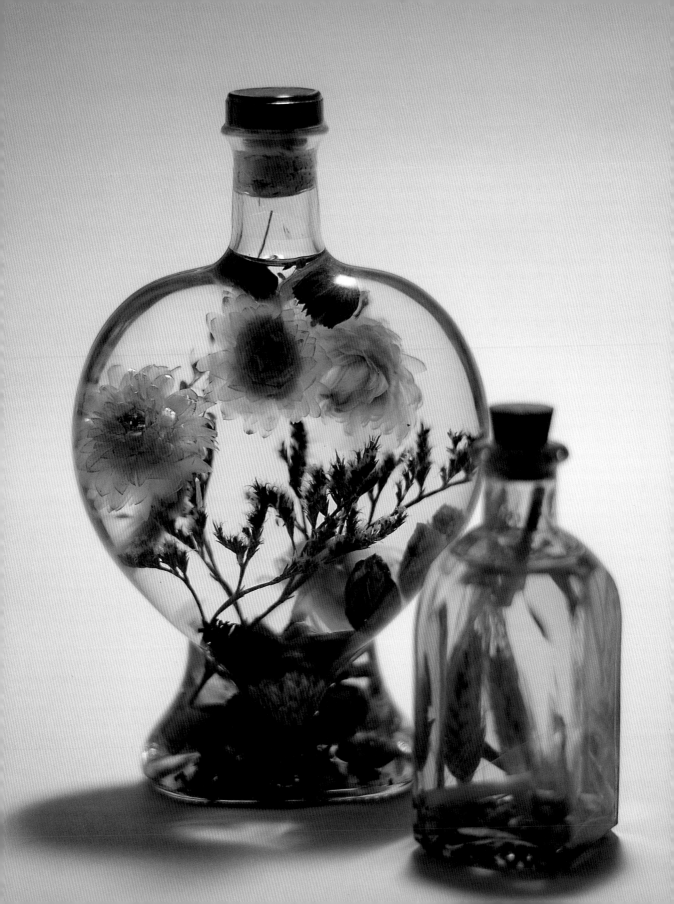

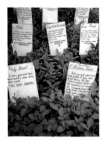

Aromatherapy

For thousands of years people have been using the oils or essences of plants to heal, soothe, and stimulate. Mesopotamian kings burned incense of cedar and myrrh to please the gods. The Babylonians used herbs for ointments, and their capital city was the center of a flourishing fragrance and spice trade.

The renowned philosopher and physician Avicenna, whose full name was Abu Ali Al-Husayn Ibn Abd Allah Ibn Sina, lived from 980 to 1037. He was court physician to Persian princes, and his *al-Quanum fi at-Tibb* (Canon of Medicine) was the primary medical text in Europe for centuries. The book was a digest of the medical and pharmacological experience of the Greeks and Persians, based on the theory of the four elements and four humors. To established theory, Avicenna added his own discoveries of tools and methods for distilling pure essential oils from plants, which he then prescribed in many of his remedies.

Modern aromatherapy began with the work of the French chemist Rene-Maurice Gattefosse, who first used the term in a 1928 treatise, *Aromatherapie.* Gattefosse stressed the superiority of natural, plant-derived oils rather than the synthetic substances that had come into vogue in the nineteenth century.

Aside from appeasing gods, inciting lovers, and alleviating ailments, fragrant oils can be added to a bath, steam vaporizer, scented candle, or massage oil to change and improve your state of mind. The oil's action works through inhalation (breathing and smell) or absorption (rubbed on the skin or soaked in).

Different oils have different properties: bergamot, chamomile, rose, and lavender are soothing; eucalyptus, rosemary, magnolia, and spearmint are stimulating. Some oils are good for softening and moisturizing like jojoba, aloe vera, wheat germ, and almond. Special stress relievers are vanilla, nutmeg, and orange.

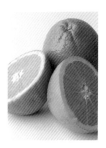 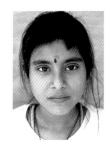 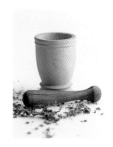

Breton Sweet Meadow Herb & Flower Bath

In summer, the fields of northern France are awash in delicate lavender and chamomile flowers, the air heavy with their scent of sweet meadows. This concoction is perfect for meditation and for soothing away stress. Basil oil is thought to soothe and promote mental acuity. Lavender, rosemary, and chamomile are known for relieving stress, relaxing muscles, and promoting healthful sleep.

3 drops lavender oil
3 drops basil oil
3 drops rosemary oil
3 drops chamomile oil

Fill a tub with warm water and add the oils. Relax.

Maharashtra Sandalwood Soak

The yellow viscous oil of the sandalwood tree has been used for centuries in perfumes and as incense in India, to promote a serene, meditative state. While traveling there, I noticed this hypnotic, sensual aroma everywhere. Eucalyptus has been used by Australian Aborigines to cure many ailments, and is especially beneficial for aching joints. This soothing combination of oils is perfect for an after-exercise soak. Eucalyptus, like many aromatherapy oils (even those made from normally digestible foodstuffs), is highly toxic if consumed. No matter how inviting these oils smell, they are never to be taken internally.

4 drops sandalwood oil
3 to 4 drops eucalyptus oil
3 drops lavender oil
3 drops rosemary oil

Combine the oils and add to a warm tub.

Regal Relaxation Bath

The finest orange blossom oil is produced in Sicily, where the trees thrive in the rich, volcanic soil. It is used by aromatherapists to ease depression and anxiety. Lavender and chamomile oils are also known for their powers to soothe.

2 drops lavender oil
2 drops orange blossom oil
2 drops Roman chamomile oil
1 drop rose oil

Combine all the ingredients. Fill the tub and get in. Never put the oil in an empty tub or directly under running water, as it will evaporate. Relax in the tub for a few minutes, then pour in the combined oils. I like to end my bath with a cooling rub with a natural sponge.

Summer Citrus Soak

This is perfect for those steamy summer nights when you can't seem to cool off. Rosemary is stimulating. Lemon and peppermint are known for their refreshing and cooling properties. Peppermint has been found in ancient Egyptian tombs dating from 1000 B.C. If you have sensitive skin or are pregnant, do not use this bath.

4 drops lemon oil
2 drops rosemary oil
2 drops peppermint oil
Juice of 1/2 lemon
2 tablespoons light safflower oil

Combine all the ingredients.
Add to a cool or lukewarm tub.

Colonial Garden Herb Bath

The herbs in this recipe could be found in the kitchen gardens of early America. They are known for their stimulating and stress-reducing properties. Cider vinegar soothes dryness and itchiness, and is used in antifatigue baths. You can use fresh herbs, if available. Put a tablespoon of water in a mortar and pestle, and crush a small handful of each herb, one at a time, to release its oils, then add the herb and water mixture to the other ingredients.

1 cup cider vinegar
1 tablespoon dried basil
1 tablespoon dried rosemary
1 tablespoon dried mint or peppermint

In a saucepan, combine vinegar with 1 cup water. Warm over low heat, but do not boil. Add the herbs and simmer for about 8 minutes. Remove from the heat and steep for several hours or preferably overnight. Strain the liquid, discarding the herbs, then bottle and label, or pour into a warm bath, sit back, and enjoy.

MASSAGE

Massage is an integral part of many health-care systems around the world. The laying on of hands, expounded by Jesus Christ, is still an important aspect of Christian faith healing. Massage is a cornerstone of Ayurveda, the techniques of which were developed in ancient India, embodying a holistic and preventive approach to medicine (see page 166). Massage has also been associated with luxuries afforded to the privileged: the esteemed Olympic athletes in ancient Greece were rubbed down with olive oil, and massage is one of the many arts the geishas of Japan offer their influential clients.

Massage is a transporting, healing experience when done properly. A fetus has the sensation of touch as early as nine weeks, making it the first of the senses to develop. The sense of touch and of being touched is appreciated on a visceral level, and an effective massage can increase one's bodily awareness. One of the primary functions of a massage is to improve blood and lymph circulation. Good circulation increases oxygen supply to the tissues, removes wastes and impurities more efficiently, and is an essential component of the immune system. Massage can relax and soothe stressed muscles, improve muscle tone, reduce fatigue, and improve bodily alignment and posture. When muscles work, chemical and electrical changes take place that alter the balance of substances in- and outside muscle cells. When this happens, muscles can contract and cramp. When muscles are tense, they constrict, often putting painful pressure on bones and nerves. Massage allows the muscles to relax, alleviating the pain and preventing potentially serious injury. Massage is often psychologically therapeutic: many people find that when they alleviate physical stress, they release emotional tensions.

Types of Massage

Many schools of massage techniques have developed over the centuries. Different types of massage are used to achieve different results. Professionals often use a combination of different techniques, adapted to each client's needs.

Swedish massage. This technique employs a system of active and passive manipulation. Swedish massage combines various hand techniques and movement of muscles and joints. It works well for improving circulation and relaxing.

Shiatsu massage. The term is short for *shiatsuryoho* ("finger-pressure therapy"). This technique, developed in Japan, is based on the theory—central to acupuncture—that there are channels of life energy (ch'i) in the body, and putting pressure on particular points along those channels or meridians helps to improve the flow of energy. Shiatsu tends to be stimulating rather than relaxing.

Sports massage. Originally developed for athletes in training, sports massage is a combination of Swedish and shiatsu techniques. Its more vigorous, performance-centered approach has found favor with a wide variety of active people who appreciate its invigorating, revitalizing effects.

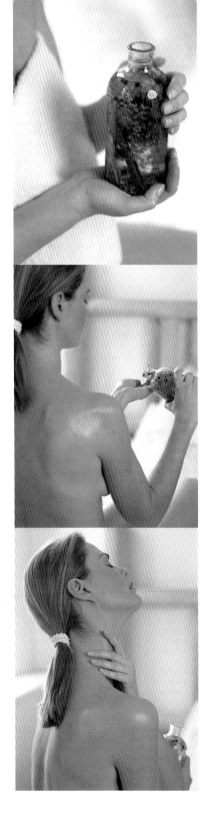

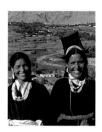

It Takes Two

Of course, you don't have to go to a professional to get a great massage, but it is necessary to have a partner. (Self-massage, possible for certain areas like the face, hands, and feet, is discussed in other chapters.)

Exotic equipment is not necessary. A floor covered by a thick, nonitchy carpet, mat, or blanket will do nicely. Don't attempt serious massage on a bed, couch, or other soft surface. When applying pressure, it's important for the body to have firm support underneath to avoid injury.

Another option is to have your massage outside on a lawn, beach, or carpet of leaves. If the terrain is wet, buggy, or irregular, you can use a massage table and still enjoy the sounds and scents of nature. If you're not outdoors, try to create in your mind all the sensations of a place you find inviting—a tropical rainforest, a sunny meadow, a secluded beach. If you like, you can play soft, unobtrusive music.

When you're getting a massage, lie down in a comfortable position, supine or prone, stretching out fully. The masseur (here the term will connote either gender) should be sure that you are comfortable, and ask if there are any special areas that he or she should concentrate on—or avoid, if there's an injury. You may or may not wish to talk during the massage, but do let the masseur know what feels good and what, if anything, does not.

Massage has always been associated with sexuality. Often it is a prelude to more intimate contact. This can be wonderful, but only if both parties agree that they want the massage to go in that direction. Whether on the giving or receiving end, you need to establish parameters. If certain things make you uncomfortable, you should ask your masseur to refrain from that sort of touching. The point of massage is to relieve tension, not increase it.

A good massage employs a variety of movements and different parts of the hands. Try long, gliding strokes; kneading, with the fingers squeezing (but not pinching) the skin and underlying muscle tissue; circular manipulation with the fingertips or knuckles.

TIPS FOR GIVING A GOOD MASSAGE

- Don't make any swift, sudden motions. Let one movement flow into the next.
- Maintain contact with the recipient. If you have to get more oil, keep one hand on the person being massaged.
- Work symmetrically. Don't overdo the right shoulder and skimp on the left.
- If you feel the recipient flinching or stiffening, ask if there's a problem; some people don't like to complain.
- Try a variety of motions, like gentle scratching or soft fingertip taps.
- Massage areas besides the back, like arms, legs, and buttocks; but keep in mind that some people are uncomfortable with touching in certain areas. When in doubt, ask.
- Always be sure to warm the oil. You can dab a little on your hand and rub it between your palms, or set the bottle in a small dish of warm water.

Massage Oils

Oils work to increase the benefits of massage. They reduce chafing and friction, and if scented aromatherapy oils are used, they can increase relaxation or invigoration, involving other senses in the process. You can mix your own essential oils, experimenting with a variety of base or carrier oils and fragrances, finding the most efficacious ones for you. Oils should be stored in a cool place in well-sealed dark bottles because exposure to heat, sunlight, and air causes unwanted changes in many kinds of oils.

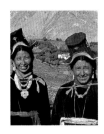

A Catalogue of Oils

These are four of the most common carrier oils, to which you can add a few drops of essential oils, which are too concentrated to be applied directly onto the skin. The basic formula is one drop of essential oil to five milliliters of carrier oil.

Almond oil

This odorless oil has been a favorite since the days of Cleopatra; the Romans used it for medicinal as well as cosmetic purposes. Almond oil was an emollient of choice because it is rich in proteins and minerals and is an excellent treatment for dry, rough, itchy skin. Almonds thrive in Mediterranean climates; their fragrant pink flowers give way to small, peachlike fruits. A member of the rose family, almond trees can grow to twenty-five feet.

Jojoba oil

Rich in vitamin E, jojoba comes from southwestern America and is used extensively by Native American peoples for all sorts of skin disorders. The oil (actually a waxy solid at room temperature) is extracted from the seeds of this shrub or small tree that belongs to the box family. Jojoba oil shares many properties with human skin oil, and can be found in cleansers, moisturizers, even anti-inflammatory preparations.

Avocado oil

A member of the laurel family native to Central and South America, avocados and their oil are used by indigenous women as a moisturizer. The rich, heavy oil is also an excellent sunblock. The fleshy green fruits are full of vitamins A and B, and lecithin, a protein with antioxidant properties that nourishes delicate skin and hair.

Olive oil

Variously a symbol of peace, purity, and victory, the olive and its products sustained much of the ancient Western world. The Mediterranean diet that relies on olive oil instead of butter is associated with a lowered rate of heart disease. Also rich in Vitamin E, olive oil is a soothing skin moisturizer with healing properties. Be sure to get oil marked "extra virgin," since this has the lowest acidity and is therefore better matched to skin pH.

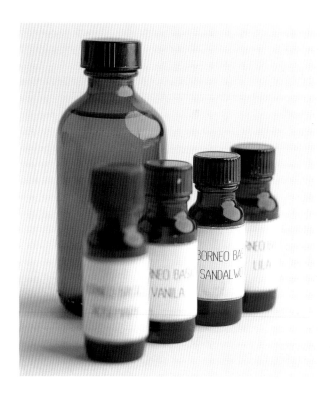

Cellulite Melter Massage

The combination of these essential oils has detoxifying properties. Geranium is known to lessen fluid retention. Rosemary oil regulates hormonal balance and breaks down fat. This massage, combined with proper nutrition and exercise, helps to combat cellulite.

2 tablespoons peanut or safflower oil
2 tablespoons olive oil
2 tablespoons almond oil
5 to 10 drops rosemary oil
5 to 10 drops geranium oil
4 drops ivy oil (optional)

Combine the oils and massage onto problem areas—hips, thighs, upper arms, and so on.

Sensual Almond Body Oil

Lanolin, the substance that keeps sheep's fleece soft and protected from the elements, can do the same for skin. Mexican women use almond oil for body massage. Almond oil was used in Imperial Rome for massage. You can add a few drops of your favorite essential oil(s). Men especially seem to love vanilla combined with the scent of almonds. I think it reminds them of Mom baking cookies.

8 to 10 tablespoons lanolin
4 tablespoons almond oil
2 to 3 drops vanilla oil

Melt the lanolin in a pan over low heat. Briskly stir in the almond oil. Let cool and add the vanilla oil.

Lover's Kiss
Massage Oil

This concoction has a sexy scent and is great for a mutual massage with your partner, or to rub on yourself after a bath or shower. Dab a bit behind the ears. Vanilla is calming, soothing, and is said to have aphrodisiacal properties. A freshly mixed batch in a special container makes a great holiday or shower gift.

1/2 cup almond oil
1/2 cup safflower oil
1/2 cup coconut oil
2 teaspoons vitamin E oil
2 teaspoons vanilla extract
2 teaspoons ground nutmeg
or cinnamon

Combine all the ingredients, and let stand for a few hours. Strain through a coffee filter into a clean bottle. Label.

Tamil Garden Soothing
Massage Oil

Patchouli comes from an East Indian shrub and has a heavy, intoxicating fragrance. In some cultures the leaves are used in religious ceremonies to bring harmony. The herbs are redolent with the scents of an exotic secret garden. Herbal essences are more readily absorbed through the skin than through inhalation.

6 to 8 tablespoons olive oil
6 to 8 tablespoons peanut oil
6 to 8 tablespoons almond oil
5 drops chamomile oil
5 drops jasmine oil
5 drops lavender oil
5 drops patchouli oil

Combine the first three ingredients to make a base oil. Put in a container, then add the essential oils, mix thoroughly, and label.

WE HAVE A SACRED RESPONSIBILITY BECAUSE OF THE SPECIAL GIFT WE HAVE, WHICH IS BEYOND THE FINE GIFTS OF THE PLANT LIFE, THE FISH, THE WOODLANDS, THE BIRDS, AND ALL THE OTHER LIVING THINGS ON EARTH. WE ARE ABLE TO TAKE CARE OF THEM.

AUDREY SHENANDOAH
Onondaga, 20th century

On the third day of the third month, in fresh weather,
The elegant women of the capital stroll on the riverbank—
Their manner regal and remote . . . What do they wear in their hair?
The hummingbird headdress with jade leaves dangling past their lips.

Tu Fu
Chinese, 8th century
from "The Elegant Women"

Chapter Three

HAIR

Shiny, healthy hair is adornment in itself. Keeping hair soft, silky, and sweet-smelling is one of the simplest and most effective ways to maintain beauty and boost confidence. For most women, however, proper hair care is no easy task. The rigors of modern life are constantly putting our hair's health in peril. Lack of sleep, stress, medications, hormonal changes, extremes of weather, and insufficient protein in the diet are some of the things that can strip the life out of hair.

The hair is a mirror of overall well-being. Often, when people are ill, their hair becomes dull and lifeless. Changes in hair can be the first signs of nutritional deficiencies. Scientists analyzing a strand of hair can discover vitamin deficiencies, exposures to toxins, and chemical imbalances—even years after the fact. Locks of President Lincoln's hair taken on his deathbed were recently tested to reveal various physiological anomalies.

While the hairdressing industry offers many products and processes to alter, control, and manage hair, some of these modern miracles can wreak havoc with your hair's health. Synthetic dyes and bleaches, permanents, and

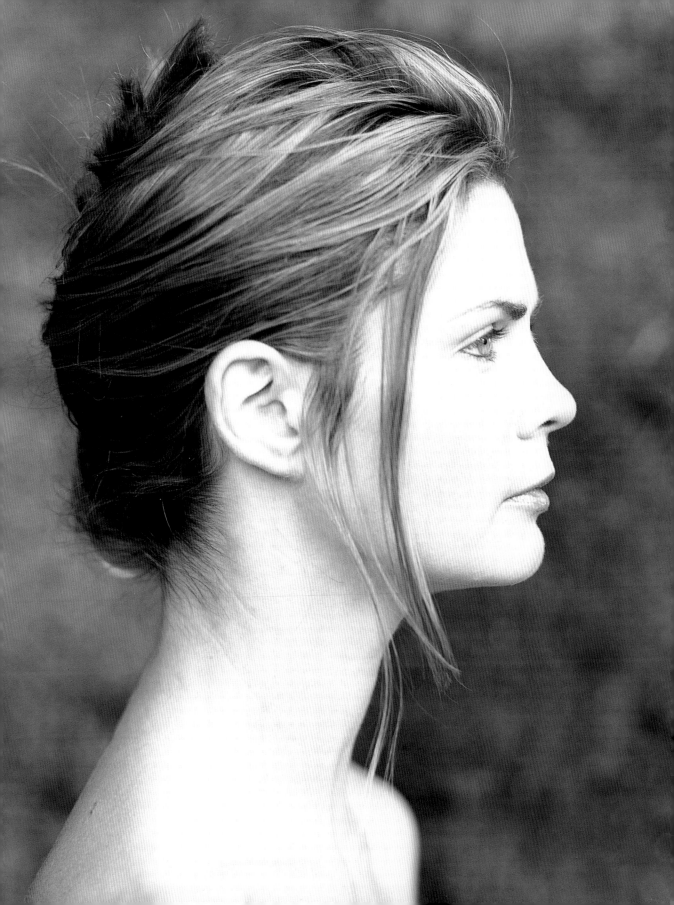

He told her all his heart, and said unto her,
There hath not come a razor upon mine head;
for I have been a Nazarite unto God from my mother's womb: if I be shaven,
then my strength will go from me, and I shall become weak,
and be like any other man.

Judges 16:17
13th to 16th century b.c.
The Bible

straightening solutions all contain harsh chemicals that drastically change the very structure of hair down to the roots. Constant overexposure to these chemicals, plus teasing, high-powered hair dryers, hot rollers, and harsh detergents weaken hair, and over time it loses its natural shine, strength, and elasticity.

Women are now seeking out natural hair-care products, or making their own. Here, you will find natural hair-care treatments and recipes that have been tested by women with all types of hair, from all walks of life, from all over the world. This chapter will allow each woman to develop a simple, practical approach to hair care.

Hair has played an important part in history and literature. Delilah sapped Samson's strength with a simple shearing while he slept. In her tenth-century masterpiece *The Tale of Genji,* Murasaki Shikibu describes the elaborate coiffures of the ladies of the Japanese court. The Brothers Grimm's tale of Rapunzel and her long hair was actually a German retelling of a French fairy tale, which was adapted from a Neapolitan collection of stories. Alexander Pope's hilarious eighteenth-century poem "The Rape of the Lock" details in mock-heroic terms the furor that erupts when an aristocrat snips a ringlet from a lady's head.

Hair is imparted with significance beyond its more prosaic functions, and through the centuries, women have discovered many ways to keep it beautiful. For example, Native Americans have been using jojoba oil for generations. Its superb conditioning qualities leave hair silky and soft. For luster and manageability, Mexican women love aloe vera and avocado oil for their hair, a combination that also acts as a partial screen against the strong Central American sun. The women of Java massage the scalp with aloe, claiming it stimulates hair follicles.

It is important to remember, however, that shiny hair is not merely a matter of finding the right shampoo. Healthy hair grows from the inside out. Since hair is a repository for, and a reflection of, all the good and ills of the body, it follows that proper nutrition is essential to keeping hair fit. Hair is nourished by the foods you eat.

Put simply, if you eat right, your hair will look better. Avoid overindulgence in sugar, caffeine, recreational drugs, and soda. Hair loss and damage due to vitamin and mineral deficiencies, sickness, and stress can often be reversed through an improved diet, plenty of water, fresh air, exercise, daily relaxation, and scalp massage.

Hair consists of protein layers called keratin. Proteins are vulnerable to surface damage, and can break down if starved of the nutrients they need. One important facet of any regmen is to provide hair with an internal source of oil and moisture.

HAIR-CARE BASICS

- Always wash your hair in warm (not hot) water, and rinse in cool water to stimulate the circulation in your scalp.

- When drying wet hair, always blot dry with a towel. Do not pull or wring. Wet hair is very fragile and vulnerable to breakage. Too much stress on wet hair can strip it of elasticity.

- Avoid blow drying whenever possible. Air dry naturally as often as you can. If you must use a blow dryer, set it on cool, and stop just before your hair is dry. There are now heat-detecting dryers on the market with sensors that automatically switch the dryer off when your hair is dry enough.

- Whether you use a blow dryer or not, flip your head upside down and fluff hair away from the scalp with your fingers, a comb, or a brush. When your hair dries, it will look fuller.

- Use a wide-toothed comb. If you have long hair, comb it in sections starting at the bottom, working up to the roots. This will avoid snarls. Hair that's properly conditioned should resist tangling. If your hair does get knotted, don't yank it with the comb. Gently pull the knot apart with your fingers, and then it comb out, always beginning at the bottom.

- Daily brushing gets rid of dandruff and stimulates the circulation of your scalp. Avoid nylon bristles; they are hard on hair, and cause split ends. Instead use a natural-bristle brush; it "understands" your hair better.

- Accessorize wisely. Just like skin, exposure to too much sun and wind can damage and dry out hair. Wear a hat or a good sunscreen on your hair. Rubber bands break hair. Opt for accessories with fabrics tied around the bands; they are gentler.

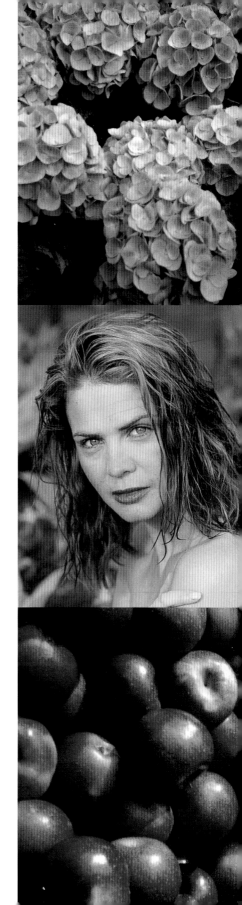

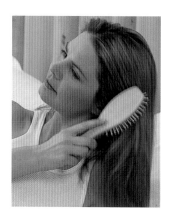

GOOD HAIR DIET

Good hair grows from a good diet. One of the most important things you can do to help grow a beautiful head of hair is drink lots of water (see page 181). Water is the essential ingredient for all of the body's systems. It maintains blood pressure and promotes circulation, which transports important nutrients to the scalp. Drink at least eight 8-ounce glasses per day (about one liter).

Here are some healthy hair choices:

- Protein-rich foods, like lean meats, poultry, fish, and legumes.

- Foods high in B vitamins, like dairy products, green leafy vegetables, legumes, eggs, whole grains and cereals, lean meats (especially liver), and yeast.

- Foods containing zinc, like lean meats (especially liver), eggs, and seafood (especially oysters).

- Moisturizing oils, like evening primrose oil and vitamin E oil (both come in easy-to-take capsules).

- Kelp, a seaweed that has a high amount of silicon, important for the roots of the hair.

Avoid:

- Too much caffeine;

- Sugar overload; and

- Megadoses of drugs, including anti-inflammatories like aspirin.

Hair Types

It is important to tailor any hair-care regimen to your individual hair type.
Most people know what type of hair they have; however, a new climate or season,
hormonal changes (during pregnancy, for instance), advancing age, even stress, can alter your
hair type temporarily or permanently. Like your complexion, you might also have combination hair.
People with long hair, for instance, often find that it is oily at the roots, dry at the ends.
In this case, you would want to give more attention to conditioning the ends,
while keeping excess oil away from the scalp.

Normal hair

Is full, glossy,
and manageable.
Keep it healthy with
gentle shampooing
every other day or so,
and conditioning
once every week.

Oily hair

Roots of the hair look and feel greasy.
If oily hair has been permed or colored,
it might still look dry at the ends.
Scalp massage is beneficial, as is regular exercise.
Cut down on fried foods.
Vitamin B is also important for oily hair.
Shampoo your hair more often,
every day or two.

Dry hair

Feels brittle, frizzy, and looks dull
and straggly, with many split ends.
Shampooing, if done correctly
and with the right products, will
remoisturize the hair.
Too much sugar in the diet
depletes vitamin B,
which is very important for healthy hair.
Weekly conditioning treatments
will return moisture to the hair
and bring it new
life and luster.

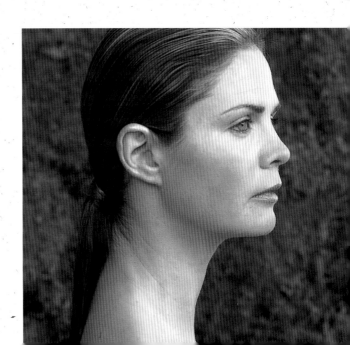

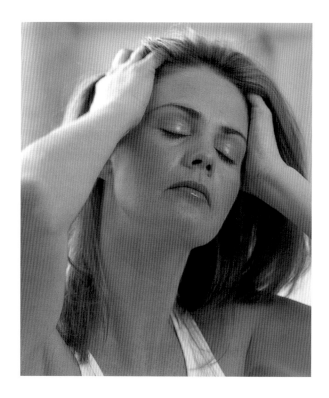

Hair Horrors & Helpers

Horrors

- Hot rollers
- High-powered hair dryers
- Chemical perms, straighteners, and relaxers
- Chemical hair colors and dyes
- Nylon-bristle brushes
- Rubber bands
- Overindulgence in sugar, caffeine, sodas, and recreational drugs
- Overexposure to sun
- Overexposure to saltwater or chlorine
- Dry heat (for example, indoors in winter)

Helpers

- Daily exercise improves oxygen flow to hair follicles.
- Massage scalp at least 3 to 5 minutes every day.
- Use a slant board for 15 minutes at least once a week to increase blood circulation.
- Rinse, alternating hot and cold water, for several minutes.
- Add aloe vera to your herbal shampoo.
- Brush hair daily with a natural-bristle brush for at least 5 minutes.

You Go to My Head: Promoting Hair Growth

Here are three activities you can do that increase circulation to the head and scalp. This helps bathe hair follicles with oxygen and nutrients, which stimulate the growth of thick, healthy hair.

Yoga headstand

The word *yoga* comes from the Sanskrit meaning "union, concentration." Yoga originated in India thousands of years ago and has since branched off into many different disciplines that promote physical and spiritual exertion and rest, leading to self-illumination (see page 157).

The yoga headstand is excellent for scalp circulation. If you haven't learned it in yoga class, you can try the shoulder stand instead. Lie on your back and lift your body and legs straight into the air and keep your feet high. Lift your buttocks off the floor and support them with your hands. Hold for a few minutes.

Slant boards

The premise of a slant board is simple: it rests at an angle from the floor, you lie on it face up with your head down toward the floor so your feet are higher, increasing blood flow to your head. Many people do exercises (like sit-ups) on a slant board because the greater resistance makes for a better workout. However, it's also a good way to just lie quietly and relax, read a book, or meditate.

A slant board reverses the effects of gravity. By doing this, you can tone and reenergize your entire body. Daily use of a slant board for 15 minutes increases circulation to the head and scalp. Slant boards can be purchased from health-food stores and athletic supply stores, or you can make one yourself out of a sturdy, sanded piece of wood.

Scalp massage

Massaging the scalp every morning for 3 to 5 minutes will stimulate hair growth, and, many doctors think, will sharpen brain function. It also gives a great feeling of well-being. Cup your hands as if you were holding a small ball. Then press down gently, but firmly on your head, and rotate your fingers in a circular motion. Move to another spot on the head, and do the same thing until your whole head feels tingly and awakened.

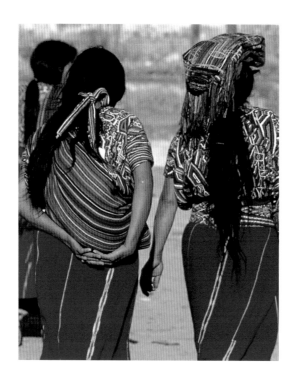

Essential Oil Aromatherapy Hair Treatments

Essential oils can boost circulation, stimulate hair follicles, and promote hair growth. They also clear and refresh the mind—so they work inside your head as well as outside. Some essential oils have therapeutic properties and can improve the health of your hair; some are used for their fragrance, to make hair smell sweet and fresh, and their soothing scents will also dissolve tension that can make hair dull. Scientists speculate that stress causes blood vessels to constrict, reducing circulation and denying hair the nutrient bath it needs to stay healthy.

Simply add a few drops of essential oil—or an infusion made from steeping herbs in boiling water—to an all-natural neutral or herbal shampoo, to the final rinse water when you wash your hair, or to one of the base oils listed below. Oils and infusions condition hair and leave it wonderfully fragrant.

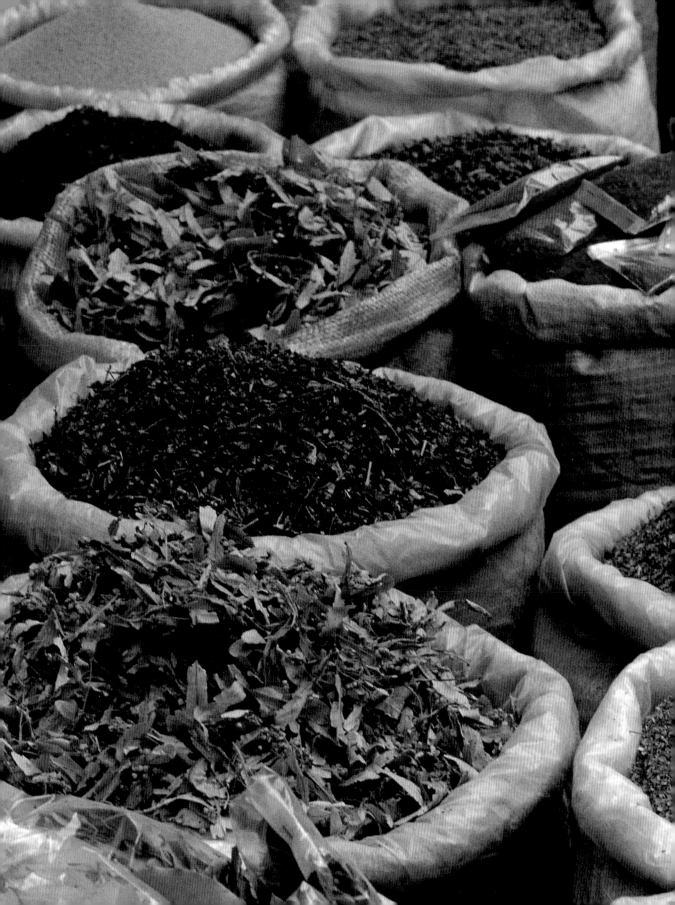

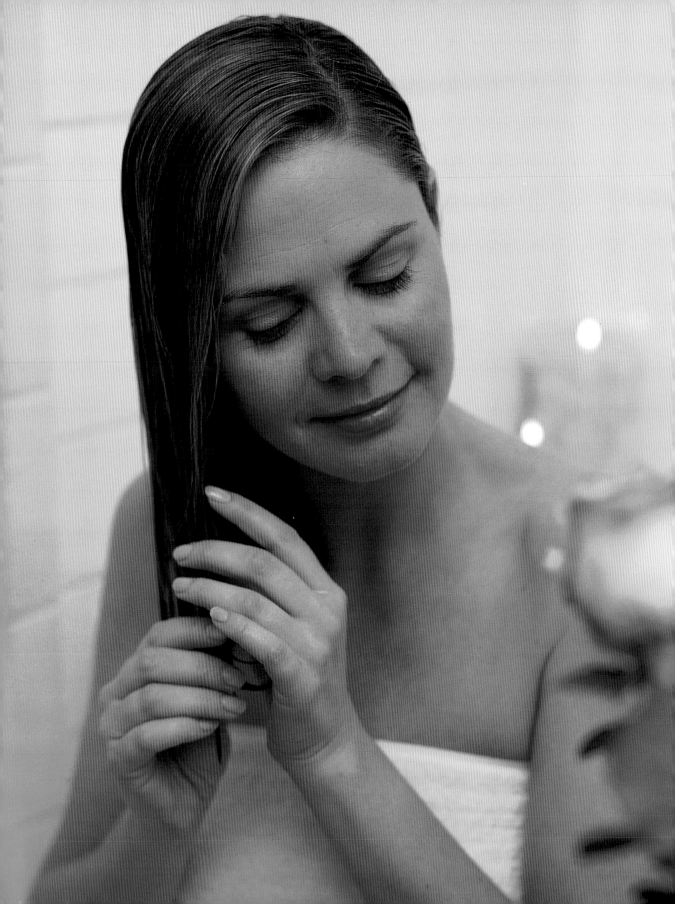

Oil and oil treatments are favored by women all over the world. All the oils mentioned are available at health-food stores.

The oils listed below can be used alone, or as a base oil mixed with a few drops of essential oil to enhance their fragrance and enriching properties: jojoba oil, evening primrose oil, castor oil, shea butter (a natural vegetable butter), almond oil, sweet almond oil, avocado oil, safflower oil, corn oil, coconut oil, and olive oil.

Try working just a few drops of nourishing oil through the ends of your hair.

For dry hair. Try jojoba oil, evening primrose oil, castor oil, almond oil, avocado oil, safflower oil, or corn oil.

For oily hair. Try castor oil, jojoba oil.

For all hair types. Sweet almond oil is an excellent all-around nourisher.

Essential Oils

Experiment with one or more of the following essential oils that suit your hair needs.

To treat dandruff. Try eucalyptus, rosemary, or sage.

To soothe scalp irritation. Try chamomile or comfrey.

To slow hair loss. Try clary sage combined with rosemary, thyme, and/or cedarwood.

To treat dullness. Try nettle, rosemary, lavender, or parsley.

For oily hair. Try lemon balm or lavender.

For dry hair. Try nettle or burdock.

For graying hair. Try sage or fo-ti root.

To add body to limp hair. Try calendula or sage.

Daily Hair Care Routine

For dry or normal hair

1 Pour a small amount of shampoo into your palms and create a lather. Then shampoo and massage into your wet hair and scalp.

2 Rinse with an herbal essential oil mixed with water to rid hair of any soap or film, then rinse with cool water.

3 Use conditioner and massage into scalp for 3 to 5 minutes, then rinse with warm water.

4 Try to give your hair a hot oil treatment every two weeks, (see page 118) or every week if your hair is severely damaged.

For oily hair

1 Pour shampoo into your palms and create a lather. Apply to wet hair and massage your scalp firmly with your fingertips; rinse with warm water and repeat.

2 Apply conditioner to the ends of your hair, or all over if your hair is damaged, and leave on for 3 minutes. Rinse with warm water.

3 Rinse with an herbal essential oil mixed with water, and massage well. Rinse with warm water.

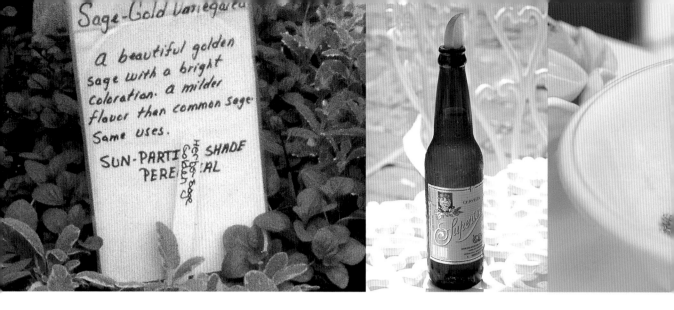

Shampoos

Shampoo cleanses the scalp and hair, loosening any dirt or oils so that they can be rinsed away. You might want to try some shampoos on the market that have natural ingredients. Have a look around your health-food store. Even some supermarkets stock natural hair-care products.

When shopping for shampoos and conditioners, it is important to read the labels. Try to find products that list recognizable ingredients—nature provides everything you need for healthy hair. Avoid products that contain a lot of ingredients whose names read like chemical formulas.

Choose products made from a natural soap, like olive oil, coconut oil, castile, or palm kernel oil. Always look for ingredients that are beneficial to your hair type. Natural ingredients are close to your hair's own makeup and rinse off thoroughly without leaving residues that attract oil and dirt. Check the resource guide at the end of this book for listings of companies that specialize in natural hair care.

Body and Beer Shampoo

Beer has been a hair-care staple since at least the Middle Ages. Most peasants in northern Europe made their own home brew and drank it like water (even young children), since drinking water could often be decidedly unhealthy. The yeast in the beer gives hair body and shine.

1 cup day-old beer (the flatter the better)
1 cup basic herbal or neutral shampoo
1 raw egg yolk (optional)

Add the beer and egg to the herbal shampoo and stir well. Pour into an empty shampoo bottle or any inexpensive squeeze bottle and shampoo as usual. (Don't worry, you won't smell like a brewery when your hair has dried.)

FOR WHOM BIND'ST THOU IN WREATHS THY GOLDEN HAIR, SIMPLY, BUT WITH SUCH STYLE?

HORACE
Roman, 1st century
from "Odes"

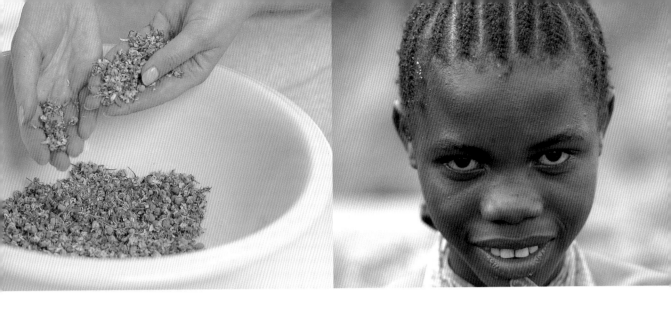

Golden Age Chamomile Shampoo (for light hair)

Chamomile comes from the Greek word *chamaimelon*, meaning "on the ground apple." It has been used for medicinal and cosmetic purposes by Mediterraneans for more than 2,000 years.

1 cup boiling water
2 tablespoons dried or fresh chamomile flowers
1/2 cup castile soap or mild shampoo
2 tablespoons glycerin
Juice of 1 lemon

Pour the boiling water over the chamomile flowers, stir, and let steep for 30 minutes to 1 hour. Strain. To the herbal water add the soap or shampoo, glycerin, and lemon juice. Stir to combine thoroughly. Pour into a clean bottle and label. Let the mixture stand for 24 hours or overnight to thicken. Shake well before using. Store in the refrigerator.

Rosemary Shampoo (for dark hair)

Rosemary is a traditional symbol for remembrance and fidelity. The ancient Greeks used rosemary as an incense at their shrines. It's great for dark hair, bringing out its natural color. You can also experiment by substituting sage or lavender for the rosemary.

4 tablespoons dried rosemary
3 pints boiling water
1/2 cup liquid castile soap or herbal shampoo
1 to 2 egg yolks (optional)

Place the rosemary in boiling water. Stir and remove from the heat. Cover and let steep for about 2 hours. Strain, and add the liquid soap or herbal shampoo to the herbal water. Stir gently until thickened. When it is cool, whisk in the eggs. Bottle, label, and let sit overnight, or for 24 hours. Shake well before using. Store in the refrigerator.

THERE'S ROSEMARY, THAT'S FOR REMEMBRANCE; PRAY YOU, LOVE, REMEMBER.

WILLIAM SHAKESPEARE
English, 16th to 17th century
from *Hamlet, Prince of Denmark*

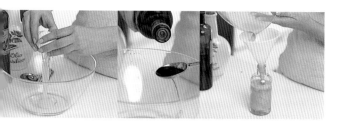

Egg and Lemon Shampoo

Famous jazz age chanteuse Josephine Baker reportedly used egg yolks to condition her hair.

2 eggs yolks
1 cup warm water
1/2 teaspoon lemon juice or apple cider vinegar

Combine all the ingredients in a blender, or whisk together thoroughly. Wet your hair with warm water and saturate with the shampoo. Massage into your scalp for a few minutes. Place one or two plastic shower caps over your head to hold in the heat for 5 to 10 minutes. Rinse with warm water.

French Lavender Shampoo

(for light hair)

While visiting the south of France I noticed the fields full of lavender. The region is a center for the perfume industry, and in spring and summer, entire valleys are planted with wonderful herbs and flowers.

1 to 2 eggs
4 tablespoons lemon juice or the juice of 2 lemons
2 teaspoons lavender water
1 drop chamomile essential oil

Combine all the ingredients and whisk until thoroughly blended. This is a soapless shampoo and will not create a lather. Gently massage the mixture into your scalp and hair. Rinse and repeat, this time leaving the mixture in your hair for about 10 minutes. Rinse with lots of warm water, then condition. You can add the ingredients to a simple all-natural castile, avocado, or coconut shampoo if you prefer more lather.

Roman Rose Shampoo

(for dark hair)

The Romans were obsessed with the rose. They bathed with roses, made fragrances with rose essence, and slept on rose petals. This is a soapless shampoo, but cleans hair and removes dirt and grime. You can add the following ingredients to a simple, all-natural castile, avocado, or coconut shampoo if you prefer more lather.

1 to 2 eggs
2 to 3 tablespoons vinegar
2 to 3 teaspoons rosewater
1 drop rose essential oil

Combine all the ingredients together. Gently massage the mixture into your scalp and hair. Rinse and repeat, this time leaving the mixture in your hair for about 10 minutes. Rinse, then condition.

Dry Shampoos

If you don't have time to shampoo, you can sprinkle these natural ingredients into your hair. Wait a few minutes, allowing dirt and oil to be absorbed, then brush through.

In the Far East, many people don't wash their hair with water. In India, they often dry brush their hair with cornmeal or some other absorbent grain meal or powder. Dry shampoos give hair a boost and maintain its acid mantle. Fuller's earth and orris powder are available at health-food stores. Use a few handfuls of one of the following—don't mix them.

Fuller's earth (natural dry clay)
Cornmeal, finely ground
Orris powder (from pulverized
Florentine iris root)
Salt (kosher or coarse salt—not
regular table salt)

Part your hair in sections. Standing outside, in a bathtub, or on old newspaper, sprinkle the dry shampoo into your scalp and hair, section by section, until your whole head is covered. Wait for 5 to 15 minutes. To absorb more dirt and oil, leave on for up to 15 minutes. Brush your hair vigorously with a natural-bristle brush.

You can also place a piece of nylon or cheesecloth over your hairbrush, with the bristles sticking through. This helps to absorb more oil and dirt.

QUICK SHAMPOO TIPS

- Alternate shampoos every few washings, because your hair goes through changes. Hair responds differently to cold and heat.
- Jojoba oil is great for damaged and dry hair. Massage 1 to 2 tablespoons into your scalp. Leave on for 1 hour or overnight, wrapped in a scarf; shampoo out.
- Shampoo that contains wheat germ oil is excellent for dry or brittle hair.
- For oily hair, shampoo once, then mix an egg with your second shampoo. The added protein gives your hair fullness and bounce.
- Soak cotton balls with apple cider vinegar, and apply to your scalp before shampooing. This is very effective for oily hair.

HERBAL HAIR TONICS AND RINSES

Hair rinses are wonderful and serve the same purpose as a toner for your face, cleansing residues and prepping hair for moisturizing. Rinses remove oils and soap films that can deprive hair of shine. Important: Do not use rinses on processed, relaxed, bleached, or permed hair. Add a few drops of the oils below to warm water and rinse with it.

For shiny dark hair. Try rosemary or sage.

To darken hair. Try rosemary, nettles, or sage.

For blond hair. Try chamomile or lemon.

For body. Try kelp or rinse with sea water.

For pH balance. Rinse with apple cider vinegar.

Herb Infusions for Hair

Put dried herbs or herbal tea bags in boiling water. Stir. Remove from the heat, cover, and allow to infuse for 2 hours.

Strain, and add the infusion to your favorite coconut, avocado, or castile shampoo.

You can improve on the following recipes by adding herbs to any of them (see below). Some of the best ingredients for a hair rinse are peppermint, rosemary, sage, coltsfoot, lemon balm, horsetail, and neutral henna (great for oily hair). You can also add a beaten egg to these recipes. For oily hair, add an egg white, which is an astringent. For dry hair, add an egg yolk. When adding egg whites or yolks, be sure to wash out the rinse—don't leave it on.

For light hair. Make an infusion of chamomile, nettle, or rhubarb root.

For dark hair. Make an infusion of rosemary, sage, or parsley.

For gray hair. Make an infusion of sage.

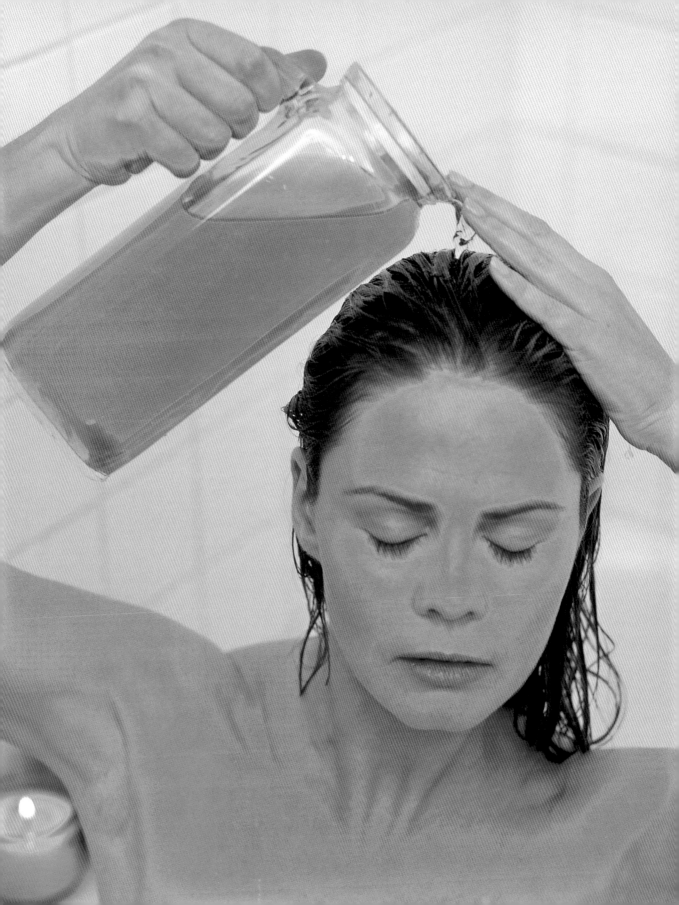

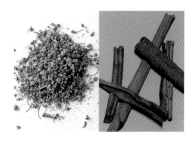

Fragrant Chamomile Infusion Rinse (for blond highlights)

Chamomile brings out the natural highlights in blond hair. It also softens the hair and adds a wonderful honeyed scent.

2 cups water
1 cup dried chamomile flowers

Boil the water and add the chamomile flowers. Remove from the heat and let steep for 1 to 2 hours. Strain. After shampooing, hold your head over a basin and pour the rinse through your hair. Try to catch the excess rinse in a basin and repeat the process. Do not rinse out the chamomile. Squeeze out the excess and towel dry. For extra lightening, let your hair dry in the sun.

Blond Bombshell Rinse

(for light hair)

Lemons are high in vitamin C and a great boost for blond hair. This is my favorite rinse to bring to the beach in the summer or on a warm-weather vacation when I want blond highlights added to my hair naturally.

1/2 cup freshly squeezed lemon juice
1/4 cup apple cider vinegar diluted with
1/2 cup water

Combine the lemon juice with the diluted vinegar. After shampooing, pour the rinse through your hair. Rinse out. For added highlights, comb through your hair, leave in, and let your hair dry in the sun.

Rhubarb Root (for light hair)

2 1/2 cups boiling water
1/4 cup chopped rhubarb

Add the rhubarb to the boiling water, remove from the heat, and let steep for 2 hours. Strain. Use the infusion as a hair rinse. You can also make this recipe as a paste by adding 1/2 cup kaolin powder to 1 cup of the infusion. Stir to combine, then add an egg yolk and a few drops apple cider vinegar to the paste. Wearing gloves, apply the paste to your hair and leave on for 20 minutes to 1 hour. Rinse thoroughly.

Rosemary Luster Rinse

(for dark hair)

Rosemary was used to prevent plague and to ward off evil spirits during the Middle Ages. Rosemary is known to strengthen and renew hair. You can also use half rosemary and half sage to make a leave-in rinse.

2 drops rosemary oil
1 to 2 cups boiling water
2 tablespoons dried rosemary

Add the dried rosemary to the water, remove from the heat, let steep for 1 hour, then add the rosemary oil.
Add to your final rinse.

Cinnamon Rinse (for dark hair)

2 cups boiling water
3 or 4 cinnamon sticks

Break the cinnamon sticks into small pieces and add to the boiling water. Let steep, cool, and strain. Rinse through your hair.

Tingling Nettle Scalp Rinse
(for dandruff)

The eau de cologne adds fragrance and acts as a preservative.

2 to 4 tablespoons dried nettle leaves
or juice (available at health-food stores)
1 pint boiling water
1/4 cup white wine vinegar
2 to 3 tablespoons eau de cologne
in your favorite fragrance

Add the nettles to the boiling water, remove from the heat, and let steep for about 1 hour, then strain the liquid. Add the vinegar and eau de cologne. Bottle and label. Massage into scalp each night.

Stimulating Hair Tonic
(for gray hair)

Here is a pleasant alternative to hair dyes that makes hair and scalp feel fresh and renewed.

2 to 4 tablespoons dried rosemary
2 to 4 tablespoons dried sage
2 cups boiling water
1/4 cup apple cider vinegar or
2 to 4 tablespoons eau de cologne (optional)

Add the rosemary and sage to the boiling water. Remove from the heat and let steep for at least 1 hour. Strain. Add the vinegar and the eau de cologne. Bottle and label. Add the tonic to your favorite shampoo or use it as a rinse.

Sage Tonic (for gray hair)

Sage is a wonderful, woodsy-smelling herb. The Romans used it to encourage conception and as a remedy for many ills.

1 cup dried sage
2 cups boiling water

Add the sage to the boiling water. Remove from heat and let steep for several hours. Strain. Holding your head over a basin, pour through your hair several times. Do not rinse out.

Tonics for Dandruff &
Itchy, Flaky Scalp

Many, if not most, people suffer from dandruff at some time. Often it flares up in winter, when the scalp is exposed to dry indoor heat. A simple way to solve the problem is to massage your scalp with one of the following: apple cider vinegar, rosewater, witch hazel, or diluted lemon juice.

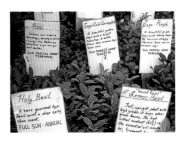

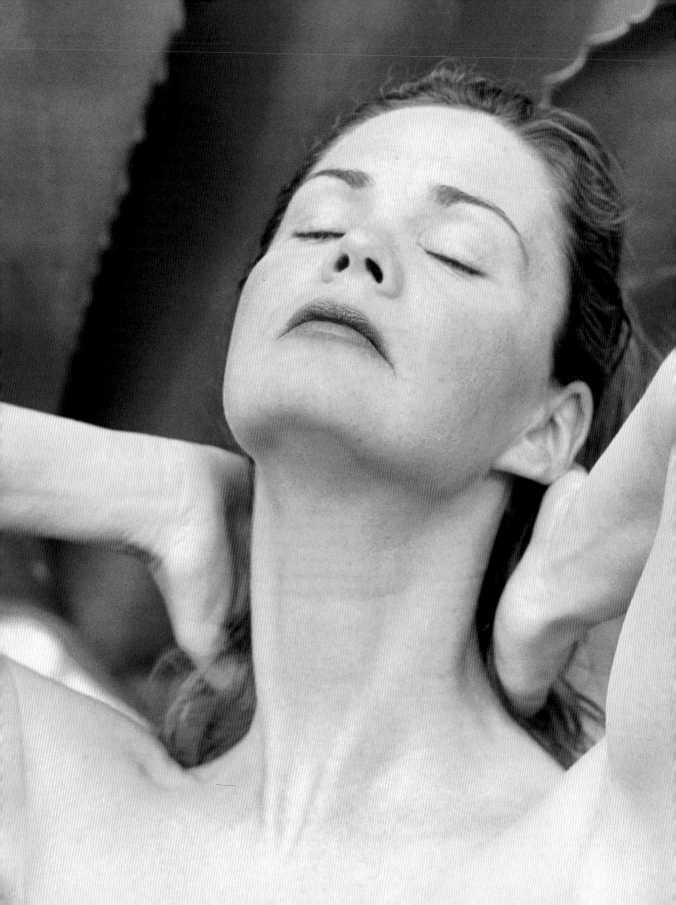

Hair Conditioning Treatments

A good conditioner nourishes your hair and acts as a detangler, making it easier to comb without breaking. It helps strengthen the hair shaft, restoring your hair's texture and luster. These are simple, gentle conditioners, and can be used every time you shampoo if you have dry hair. If your hair is oily, use these conditioners on the ends only; use all over if your hair is very damaged. You need only a quarter-sized dab: distribute it through your hair with your fingers or a wide-toothed comb.

Phillip Kingsley's Protein Conditioner (for African American hair)

This sinfully rich conditioner comes from my friend, Phillip Kingsley, who has a devoted following of celebrities at his salons in New York and London. He has been a trichological consultant—studying the physiology of hair—since 1955.

2 eggs
2 ounces cream cheese
1/2 cup heavy cream
2 tablespoons castor oil
2 tablespoons unsalted butter
2 tablespoons purified water
Juice and pulp of a medium-sized grapefruit

Combine all the ingredients together in an electric blender until smooth. Refrigerate overnight. Part your hair into sections, and apply the mixture, one section at a time, starting at the scalp and working down through the hair. Gently massage your scalp with your fingertips for about 5 minutes. Rinse out. If your hair is very dry, wrap with clear plastic, cover with 2 shower caps, and leave on overnight.

Phillip Kingsley's Conditioner (for Asian hair)

This preshampoo treatment works very well on Asian hair. This can be whipped up right in your kitchen.

2 eggs
1 ounce castor oil
1/2 ounce olive oil
1 ounce melted unsalted butter
2 ounces plain yogurt
1 banana
Juice of 1 lemon

Combine all the ingredients in a blender until creamy. Refrigerate overnight and use as necessary. Apply to the hair in sections, making sure you apply to the ends. Massage into the scalp for a few minutes. Leave on for 20 minutes, rinse out, then shampoo and condition with your regular products.

Phillip Kingsley's Conditioner

(for caucasian hair)

This preshampoo treatment can also be whipped up in your kitchen.

2 eggs
4 ounces cottage cheese
1 ounce melted unsalted butter
1 ounce purified water
Juice from a medium-sized grapefruit

Combine all the ingredients in a blender until creamy. Refrigerate overnight. Separate hair into sections and apply mixture to one section at a time, starting at the scalp and working your way down through the length of the hair. Gently massage the scalp with your fingertips for 5 minutes. If hair is very dry, wrap it in clear plastic, cover with 2 shower caps, and leave on overnight.

Caribbean Queen Conditioner

Many women of color from the Caribbean use this mixture to protect their hair from the dry climate.

1 or 2 eggs
1 tablespoon olive oil
1 tablespoon glycerin
1/2 cup purified water
1 teaspoon apple cider vinegar

Combine all the ingredients, and whisk thoroughly. After shampooing, massage the conditioner through your hair and cover with a plastic shower cap. Leave on for at least 15 to 20 minutes. Rinse thoroughly.

Galilee Almond Oil Conditioner

In Hebrew, the word for almond is *shaqedh,* "the wakeful tree," since it is often the first to bloom in spring. Originally from Persia, the almond was brought to Palestine centuries ago. It is mentioned throughout the Bible, and the Israelites used its flowers as motifs for decorative and ceremonial objects.

This wonderful conditioner can be used after shampooing or right before showering, rubbed all over your hair and body.

1 cup plain yogurt
1 tablespoon honey
1 tablespoon almond oil
1 tablespoon wheat germ

Combine all the ingredients in a bowl. Slather all over your hair, wait a few minutes, then rinse with warm water.

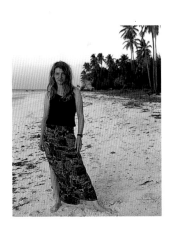
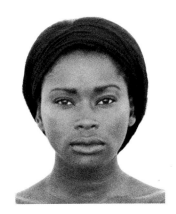
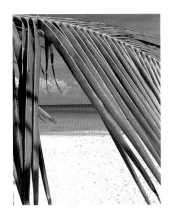

Tahitian Cocoa Butter Conditioner

While traveling in Tahiti, I learned that the women there use cocoa butter to keep their hair and skin soft. It helps protect against the harmful effects of the strong tropical sun. Cocoa butter is actually a fatty wax that is obtained from the seeds of the cocoa plant. Many of my friends rub it on trouble spots during pregnancy to prevent stretch marks. Make sure you use 100 percent cocoa butter, available in most health-food stores or drugstores.

1/2 cup safflower oil or sweet almond oil
1 tablespoon cocoa butter
1 tablespoon lanolin or soya margarine

Place the oil and lanolin in a double boiler. Melt, and add the cocoa butter. Stir until all the ingredients are completely dissolved. Remove from the heat and whisk until cool. Place in a jar and label. This is a great preshampoo conditioner. Use on very dry hair or hair that has been overexposed to the sun. Massage into your scalp and on ends of your hair. Wrap your head in a warm towel or plastic wrap and leave on for 1 to 2 hours, then shampoo out.

THERE IS NO EXCELLENT BEAUTY THAT HATH NOT
SOME STRANGENESS IN THE PROPORTION.

FRANCIS BACON
English, 16th century
from "Of Beauty"

HOLLYWOOD HAIR CONDITIONERS

Many well-known film actresses swear by this pair of simple treatments. Hollywood hair often needs extra care since it takes a beating from constant styling, coloring, and exposure to hot lights. These are also favorites among my African-American friends, great for sheen and manageability.

- Wet your hair. Pat with a towel to remove excess water, then apply 3 to 4 tablespoons of mayonnaise. Wrap your hair in a towel for about 30 minutes. Rinse, then shampoo.

- Combine 2 to 3 tablespoons of yogurt with 1 egg. Wet your hair, and massage the conditioner into your scalp. Wrap your hair in a towel for about 30 minutes. Rinse, then shampoo.

Yucatan Beer and Jojoba Conditioner

While I was visiting the Yucatan in Mexico I ran out of hair conditioner. I bought some jojoba oil, which is sold everywhere there, and mixed it with a little Mexican beer. My hair came out silky and shiny and full of body. Jojoba comes from the jojoba bean that grows wild in the desert. Many Mexican women have long, gorgeous dark hair, and use jojoba often as a hair and skin conditioner.

1 cup warm Mexican beer
1 teaspoon jojoba oil
1 egg yolk (optional)

Whisk together the beer, jojoba oil, and egg yolk. Massage the mixture into your scalp and through your hair. Rinse thoroughly with warm water

QUICK HAIR CONDITIONING TREATMENTS

These ingredients can be applied directly to your hair. You can choose one or combine several. Use 1/2 cup or less, depending on the length of your hair. Leave the conditioner on for 10 to 15 minutes, then shampoo out. It's great to use once a week.

For normal hair. Try mayonnaise, eggs, plain yogurt, olive oil, castor oil, and jojoba oil.

For dry hair. Try avocado, mayonnaise, banana, and coconut oil.

For oily hair. Add 1 to 2 teaspoons of lemon juice or apple cider vinegar to any one of the following: eggs, plain yogurt, olive oil, castor oil, or jojoba oil.

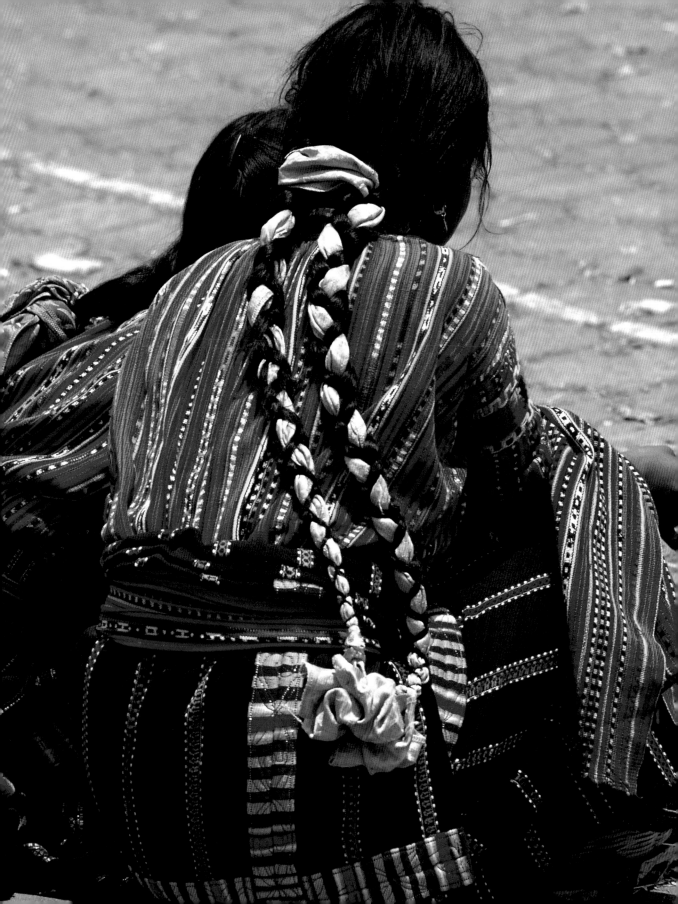

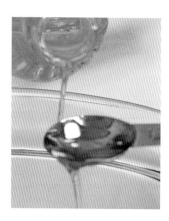

HOT OIL TREATMENTS

Hot oil treatments are great for treating dry, overworked, or lifeless hair. The heat thins the oil, helping it to better penetrate the hair shaft to repair damage. Your hair will benefit from this deep conditioning every 2 to 4 weeks—or every 2 weeks if your hair is very damaged. Do not apply hot oil treatments more frequently than every 2 to 4 weeks. Too much of a good thing can damage hair.

Warm the oil until it is well heated, but not so hot that you cannot touch it. Apply the oil sparingly. If you pour oil all over your head, it might take several washings over several days to get it out, depending on your hair length. If you have short hair, you should use no more than 1 tablespoon; if you have long hair, use 1 to 2 tablespoons. Massage into your hair, working out from roots to ends.

Cover your hair in plastic wrap, then cover with either two plastic shower caps or warm, moist towels. Leave on for about 20 minutes to deeply condition. If you soak in a warm bath while conditioning with oils, the added heat and steam will help the oil penetrate the hair. Shampoo and condition.

If your hair is very dry or severely damaged, leave on overnight. In the morning, shampoo out and finish with your favorite conditioner. Your hair will be noticeably shinier and softer.

Aromatherapy steam conditioning also encourages hair growth and helps to rejuvenate dull, lackluster, dry hair. Oils with stimulating properties that are especially effective as steaming conditioners include mint, ginger, fennel, lavender, rosemary, sage, and chamomile.

Combine one or more essential oils with a carrier oil, like jojoba or olive oil, apply to hair, then steam by sitting in a hot tub or steam room. The added heat from the steam increases the absorption of the oils.

Apennine Olive Oil Treatment

Some of the finest olive oil in the world comes from the hilly regions of central Italy. This oil has a deep, rich green color and a characteristic nutty fragrance. Use olive oil sparingly or you will have difficulty rinsing it out.

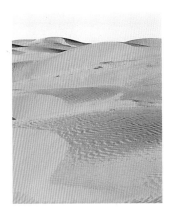

1 to 2 tablespoons Tuscan or
Umbrian olive oil
1/2 cup apple cider vinegar

Warm the olive oil. Gently massage it into your scalp and work it through your hair to the ends. Wrap your head with 2 plastic shower caps or a hot, wet towel. Leave on for 15 to 20 minutes, then wash your hair with an herbal shampoo. Apply the shampoo without adding water to cut down on the oil. Rinse with apple cider vinegar.

High Desert Hair Moisturizing Treatment

Although its ingredients are native to the Southwest, this recipe comes from Barbara Close of Naturopathica, a holistic health center in East Hampton, New York. The rich, hydrating jojoba oil attracts and retains moisture.

1 tablespoon jojoba oil
1 tablespoon sesame oil
1 teaspoon avocado oil
1/2 teaspoon honey
3 drops geranium oil
6 drops evening primrose oil
or 2 drops carrot seed oil

Combine all the ingredients in a heat-proof bowl, and set in a partially filled pot of water over low heat. When the oils are warm, gently massage into scalp and throughout your hair. Cover with a plastic shower cap and leave on for about 10 minutes. Shampoo and condition as usual.

WRAP

Lavender & Rosemary Treatment

This recipe smells heavenly. The sweet lavender complements the spicy, woodsy rosemary.

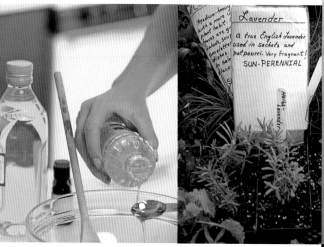

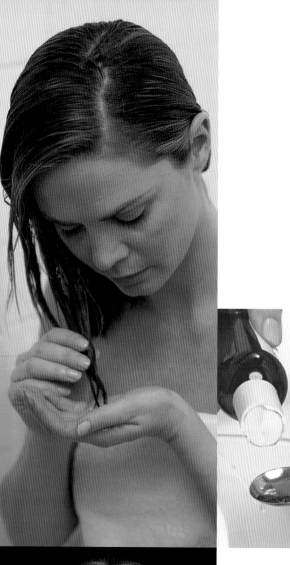

1 to 2 tablespoons olive oil
1 drop lavender oil
2 drops rosemary oil

Combine all the ingredients, and rub the mixture into the ends of your hair if they're especially dry, or massage into your scalp. Wrap in a hot towel or cover with a plastic shower cap. Let the oil soak into your hair for about 1 hour, then wash with a natural shampoo and rinse.

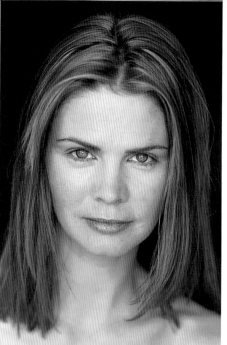

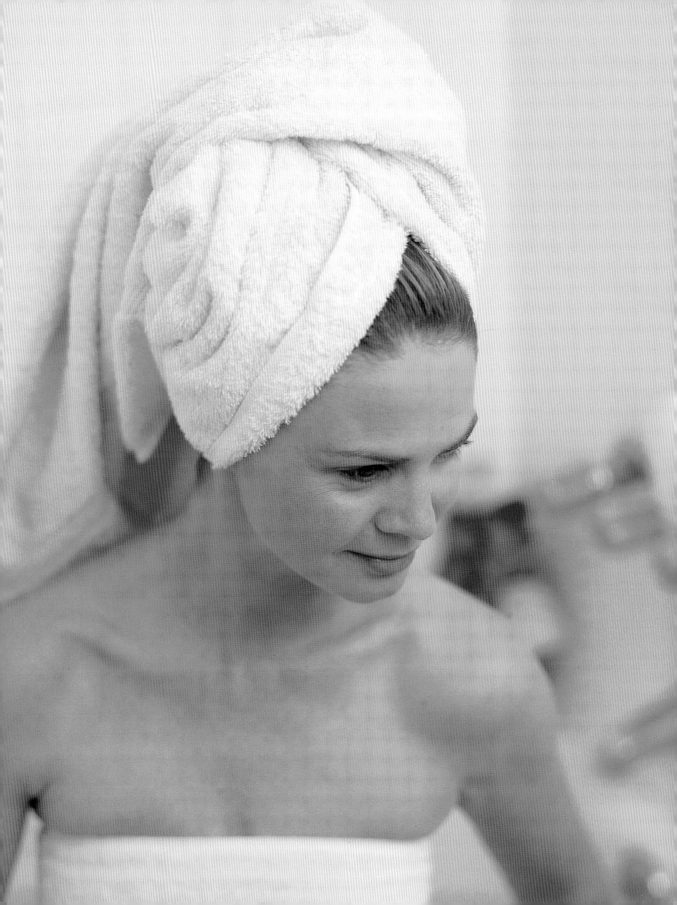

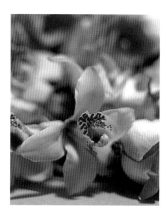

Hot Sandalwood Treatment

3 tablespoons sesame oil or olive oil
2 drops rose oil (optional)
3 drops sandalwood oil

Combine all the ingredients and rub the mixture into the ends of your hair if they're especially dry, or massage into your scalp. Let the oil soak into your hair for 15 to 20 minutes, then wash with a natural shampoo and rinse.

Ylang-Ylang Hair Treatment
(for dry hair)

Women of Tahiti mix coconut oil with a few drops of ylang-ylang to use on their hair.

Ylang-ylang has a delicious scent; it's also an aphrodisiac and its scent is said to induce euphoria.

1 to 2 tablespoons sesame oil or olive oil
1 teaspoon honey
1 egg
1 drop ylang-ylang oil

Warm the sesame oil slightly over very low heat. Remove from the heat, let stand just until it's cool enough to touch, then combine with the remaining ingredients, stirring until thoroughly blended. Massage the mixture into your scalp and through your hair. Wrap your hair in plastic wrap or a warm towel and leave on for 20 to 30 minutes. Shampoo and condition as usual.

SIMPLE OIL TREATMENTS

1 For damaged or lackluster hair, try rose hip seed oil (available at health-food stores or by mail order). Pour a small amount into your palms and massage through your hair. Style as usual.

2 Warm jojoba oil, then massage into your scalp and hair ends. Leave on for at least 1 hour, then wash out. This treatment is good for dry hair.

3 Combine 1 to 2 tablespoons olive oil with 1 to 2 drops of an essential oil of your choice, depending on your hair type (see page 97). Heat the oils and massage through your hair, then wrap in plastic wrap and a warm towel to lock in the heat. Leave on as long as you can—overnight, if possible.

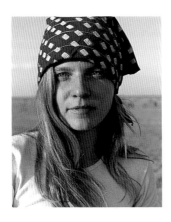

NATURAL HAIR COLORING

Changing your hair to a different shade, or enhancing your own natural color, is a great way to give yourself a boost. While commercial hair-coloring products are often harsh and harmful, there are natural alternatives that can actually improve your hair's health.

Henna has been used for thousands of years as a hair-coloring agent, and also for body painting and nail coloring (see box on Mehndi, page 135). Henna is a natural, noncarcinogenic substance derived from the leaves of a tropical shrub or small tree. A member of the loosestrife family, which includes primroses, henna is a leafy plant with clusters of fragrant white flowers.

Henna hair coloring lasts three to six months, then gradually washes out. You can experiment with different types of henna to achieve the color of your choice: brown, black, auburn, or red. My hair is on the light side, so I tried chamomile henna and was very happy with the results. It brightened my hair and made it incredibly soft and shiny.

Always test the henna on a few strands in the back of your head to make sure the color is to your liking. Sometimes henna-colored hair goes through an adjustment period for about two days after the first application; it can appear brassy at first, but the color should soon settle into a more natural shade.

If you are coloring your hair for the first time, professional colorists advise going easy. They suggest leaving the color on your hair for half the time suggested in the directions. If the color isn't as strong as you like, you can always repeat the process. It's easy to add more color; it's much more difficult to fix color that has been overdone. Starting slowly allows you more control over the results.

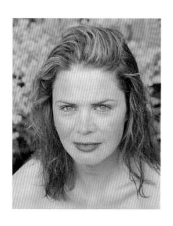
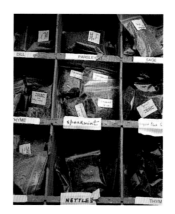
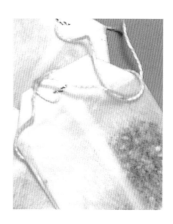

Basic Henna Coloring

The higher the ratio of henna powder to water, the deeper the color you will get. Since henna can be drying, rub a little oil (safflower works well) into your scalp before using it. Always wear gloves when working with henna, and do not use metal bowls or metal utensils with henna. Wrap an old towel around your shoulders so you don't soil your clothes.

1/2 to 1 cup pure henna powder (your choice of color)
1/2 to 1 cup boiling water
1 to 3 teaspoons apple cider vinegar

Start with clean, dry hair. Place henna in a plastic or ceramic bowl. Slowly add the boiling water to the henna, stirring the mixture until it is thickened to about the consistency of wallpaper paste. Stir in the vinegar

With hair clips, separate your hair into inch-wide sections. Wearing gloves, dip a paintbrush or your fingertips into the henna and cover your entire head, section by section. Massage to distribute the henna evenly throughout your hair. Cover with plastic wrap or a shower cap. Try to keep your head warm by sitting in the sun or wrapping a warm, wet towel around the covering.

The longer you wait before rinsing out the henna, the darker the color will be: leave it in for at least 45 minutes, or up to 3 hours for dark coloring. Rinse your hair until the water runs clear. Wash with mild shampoo.

Queen of Sheba Henna

(for dark hair)

The Queen of Sheba is reported to have been a henna devotee, using it to add richness to her natural highlights.

1 to 2 cups boiling water
1/2 cup pure neutral henna powder
3 tea bags
(Ceylon or black tea)

Make a strong tea by placing the tea bags in the boiling water and allowing them to steep for a few minutes. Follow the directions in the basic henna recipe above, substituting the tea for the plain water added to the henna powder.

Midnight Sun Fragrant Chamomile Paste (to lighten hair)

Swedish women soak chamomile flowers, then extract the blue-green–colored juice and rinse it through their hair.

2 to 4 tablespoons chamomile flowers
1 pint boiling water
1/2 to 1 cup kaolin
1 egg yolk (optional)

Put the chamomile flowers in a heat-proof bowl and cover with the boiling water; let steep for about 20 minutes. Strain. Combine 1 cup of the infusion with the kaolin and egg yolk, and stir to form a paste. Apply to hair, distributing the paste evenly, and leave on for 20 to 60 minutes—the longer you leave it on, the lighter the hair gets. Shampoo out.

Fresh Sage Darkener (for gray hair)

This is a gentle way to gradually color gray hair; because it's meant to be used over a period of days or weeks, you can control how much gray you want to cover.

3 to 4 tablespoons dried sage
1 pint boiling water
4 teaspoons rum
1 ounce glycerin
A few drops vitamin E

Put the sage in a heat-proof bowl and cover with the boiling water. Cover the bowl and let steep for 2 hours. Strain and add the rum, glycerin, and vitamin E. Bottle and label. Rub the darkener into your scalp with a cotton pad each day until the desired shade is achieved.

HAIR TIPS

1 Before shampooing, massage plain yogurt into your scalp and leave on for 20 minutes to help eliminate dandruff.

2 Mix 1 egg with your second shampoo for bounce and added protein.

3 A few drops of ylang-ylang oil with warmed coconut oil or sesame oil is an effective treatment for dry hair.

4 For African-American women who have relaxed hair: wrap your hair in a silk scarf at night. Cotton pillowcases can be rough on hair, causing breakage.

5 For styling, use alcohol-free gels instead of hair sprays, which can damage your hair and pollute the environment.

6 Club soda is a great hair rinse.

7 Rinsing with apple cider vinegar or sea water makes your hair thicker and fuller.

8 Lemons squeezed over your hair on a sunny summer day bring out your hair's natural highlights.

9 Combine 2 teaspoons sweet almond oil with 4 tablespoons castile shampoo and use as a conditioner and detangler.

10 Rinse with flat champagne to bring out blond highlights.

11 Flat beer is a great settling lotion that adds body and shine; comb through hair, let dry, then comb out.

12 If you don't have time to wash your hair, cut a square from an old pair of pantyhose and run it through the bristles of your hairbrush to absorb and remove dirt and grime; brush until your hair looks clean.

Chapter Four

HANDS & FEET

Graceful, delicate hands have long held a fascination for both sexes, and soft, supple feet are considered erogenous zones in many cultures. Anyone who has experienced a soothing hand massage or vigorous foot rub instantly appreciates that these are very hard-working extremities that could truly benefit from careful attention now and then. Hands are used for everything from slinging a sledgehammer to caressing a child. Feet support your entire body and the weight of the world beneath, and sometimes travel a rocky road. Hands and feet take a beating in any society: grinding flour for bread or matzoh or tortillas, climbing to mountain pastures, plucking chickens, chasing children, tanning hides, planting rice, walking to market, mending fishing nets, changing tires, dancing the night away.

Fortunately, hardworking women need not have the hands and feet to show for it. Since many chores that in traditional cultures are considered women's work are also very tough on hands and feet, throughout the centuries women

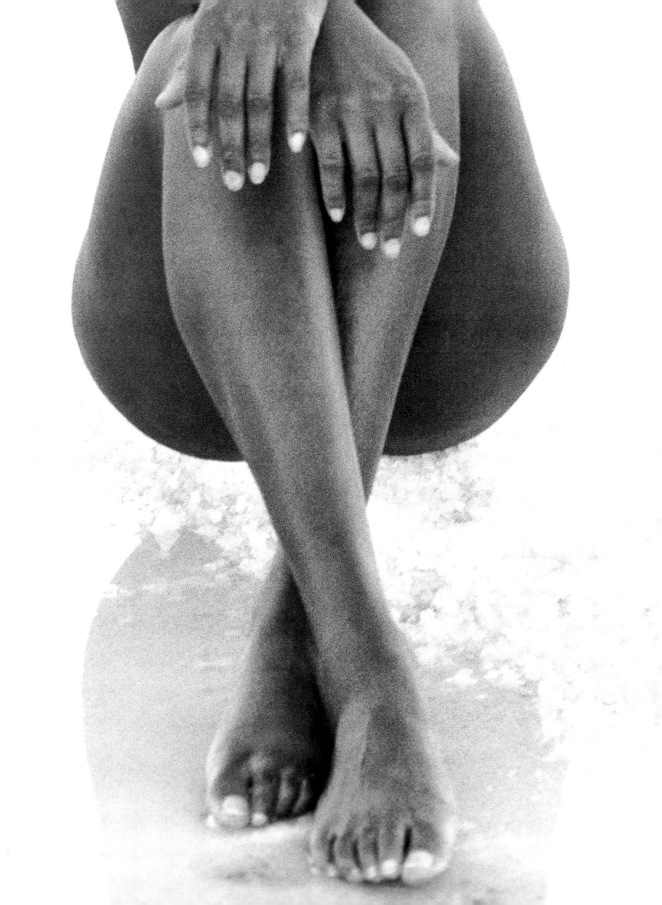

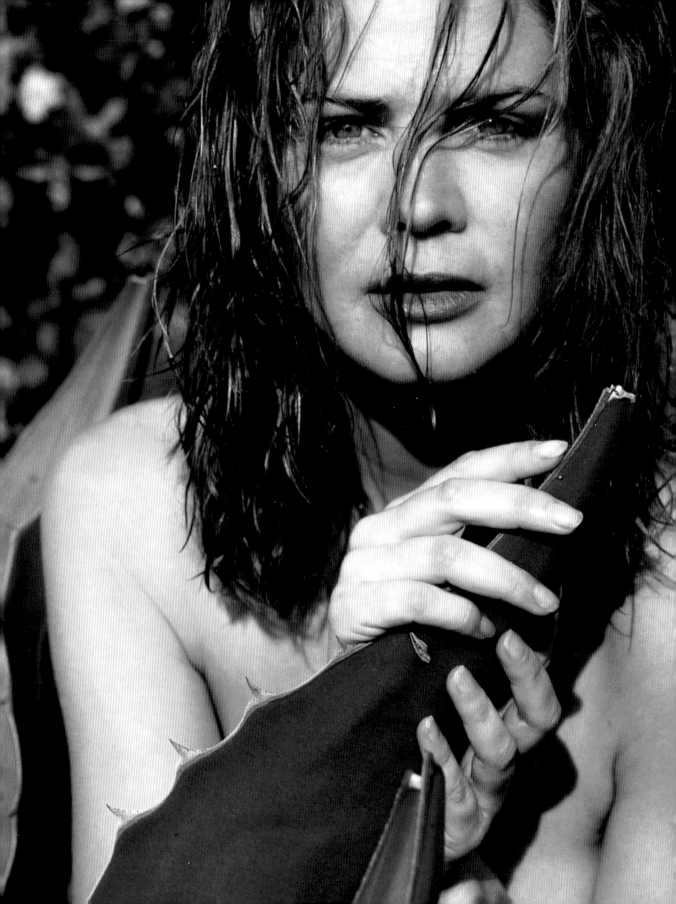

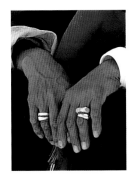

have developed simple, effective ways to smooth calluses, moisturize dryness, and eliminate roughness. Spanish women often protected their hands by wearing gloves lined with pomade to bed. Australian aboriginal tribespeople use tea tree oil to protect their feet while walking about the dry outback.

Nutritional strategies are also effective in promoting the health of skin and nails; the condition of your nails can serve as an early-warning system signaling changes in health. Protein, vitamin, and mineral deficiencies can make nails brittle and breakable. Hormonal changes also affect the nails; for instance, many women find that their nails and cuticles change at around the same time during each monthly cycle. One friend of mine says that her nails got ragged and chipped when she was pregnant.

Some holistic doctors diagnose health and illness by examining the feet. Major energy channels end at the feet. The practice of reflexology focuses massage on different areas of the feet to alleviate ills in the body's limbs and internal organs (see reflexology box, page 153), and many important acupuncture points are located on the feet, including one very useful one that is said to induce labor. In Judeo-Christian writings, there are many examples of saints and priests anointing the feet of the poor as an act of grace and humility.

Hands that look like they never did a day's work have historically been a calling card of members of the leisure classes. In western Europe, the ideal hand would have been smooth, untanned, with long, graceful "aristocratic" fingers. Queen Elizabeth I was very proud of her slender fingers, and in royal portraits they can be seen prominently displayed, holding various objects. In the novels of Jane Austen, delicate feminine hands play the pianoforte, arrange flowers, paint china, and do decorative needlework; those hands are never seen performing manual labor or even dressmaking, which was considered to be a working-class activity.

Plantation belles of the antebellum South shielded their hands from the freckle-causing sun by wearing gloves and carrying parasols, and

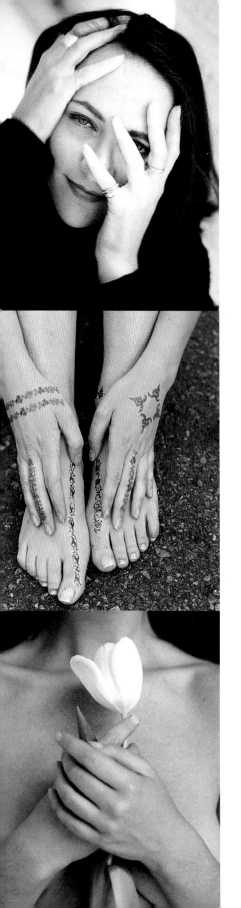

THE DELICATE HANDS OF A GIRL
BELONG TO THE INNER ROOM;
TRAINED IN THE LUTE, SHE
WOULD NEVER LEAVE THE HALL ALONE.
NOT HAVING SEEN THE FRONTIER
ROAD UNDER DUSTY CLOUDS,
HOW COULD SHE KNOW THE MUSIC
THAT BREAKS ONE'S HEART?

OU-YANG HSIU
Chinese, 11th century
from "Song of the Radiant Lady"

they softened their hands with buttermilk rinses.
When Scarlett O'Hara, gorgeously decked out
in the infamous curtain dress, pays a call on
Rhett Butler in an Atlanta jail, one look at her
cotton-picking, rough hands tips him off that
her lady-of-leisure airs are a sham.

Having strong, long nails is a visible sign of
health and prosperity. Manicuring and coloring
the nails are nothing new. Myrrh has been used
by African peoples to strengthen their nails for
thousands of years. Egyptians dipped their
fingertips in orange henna to decorate the nails.
In some places, long nails are symbols of power:
members of the Chinese nobility grew their
fingernails to absurd lengths, and decorated
them with jewel-encrusted nail guards.

130

HAND TREATMENTS AND MOISTURIZERS

What better way to show off those lovely baubles (and maybe encourage that kiss, too)
than with smooth-as-silk hands? So much of what women do with their hands saps moisture
from the skin: contact with harsh detergents, chlorine, nail polish remover, hot sun, cold wind,
and dry heat can ravage the skin, causing dryness, cracking, ridges, and wrinkles.

These recipes are delightfully soothing and help return moisture to overtaxed hands. As you apply them, take a few moments to give yourself a hand massage. Work the ingredients into your palm and the back of your hand. Start at the base of each finger and work up to the tip. Be sure to get in between the fingers, where the skin is usually most dry.

Many of these recipes work especially well if you apply the treatment, cover with cotton gloves, and leave on overnight. Be sure to use 100-percent cotton (not synthetic) gloves, as they allow air to pass through the fibers so your hands can breathe.

Enriching Hand Oil

The word sesame is from the Greek word meaning "from India," where the plant originated. In Asia, sesame is endowed with aphrodisiacal properties. This blend of oils, glycerin, and honey is excellent for chapped hands. Vitamin E is an all-around skin nourisher.

1 tablespoon olive oil
1 tablespoon sesame oil
1 tablespoon almond oil
1 teaspoon vitamin E oil
(or the equivalent in capsules)
1/2 tablespoon glycerin
1 teaspoon clear honey

In a small saucepan, over low heat, warm the honey until it's runny (but don't let it boil), then add the oils, vitamin E, and glycerin. Stir until thoroughly combined, place in a jar or pot, and label. Before going to bed, rub this rich, hydrating oil into your hands and nails for several minutes. Put on a pair of cotton gloves and leave on overnight.

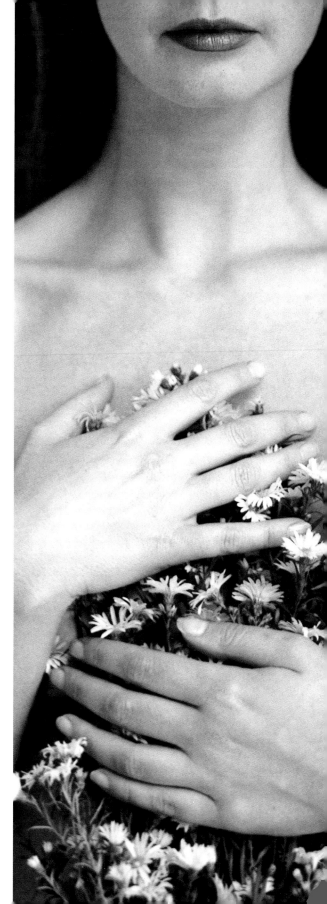

Banana Split Hand Softener

This is another of my favorite treatments for rough, chapped hands. Bananas originated in West Africa, where they were referred to as "God's gift to man." Banana plants are herbs, cousins of ginger, and the fruit is rich in vitamins and minerals, especially potassium.

1/2 ripe banana
1/2 teaspoon of honey
1 to 2 teaspoons unsalted butter
A few drops vitamin E (optional)

Combine all the ingredients until the mixture is creamy. Smooth the softener all over your hands. Put on a pair of cotton gloves and leave on overnight.

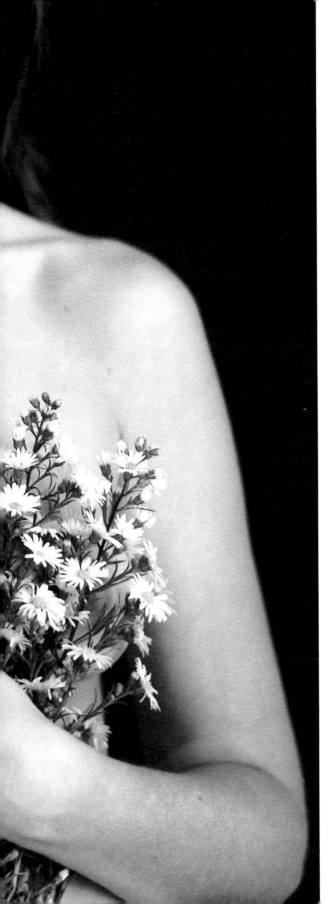

Rajasthan Oatmeal Hand Treatment

This is based on a recipe I acquired during my travels to northern India, where women commonly use oatmeal or almond meal to soften their hands.

2 tablespoons oatmeal or almond meal
1 egg yolk
1 tablespoon honey
A few drops milk
A few drops cider vinegar

Combine all the ingredients to form a thick paste, adding just enough milk and vinegar to moisten the mixture. Apply to your hands, put on a pair of cotton gloves, and leave on overnight.

133

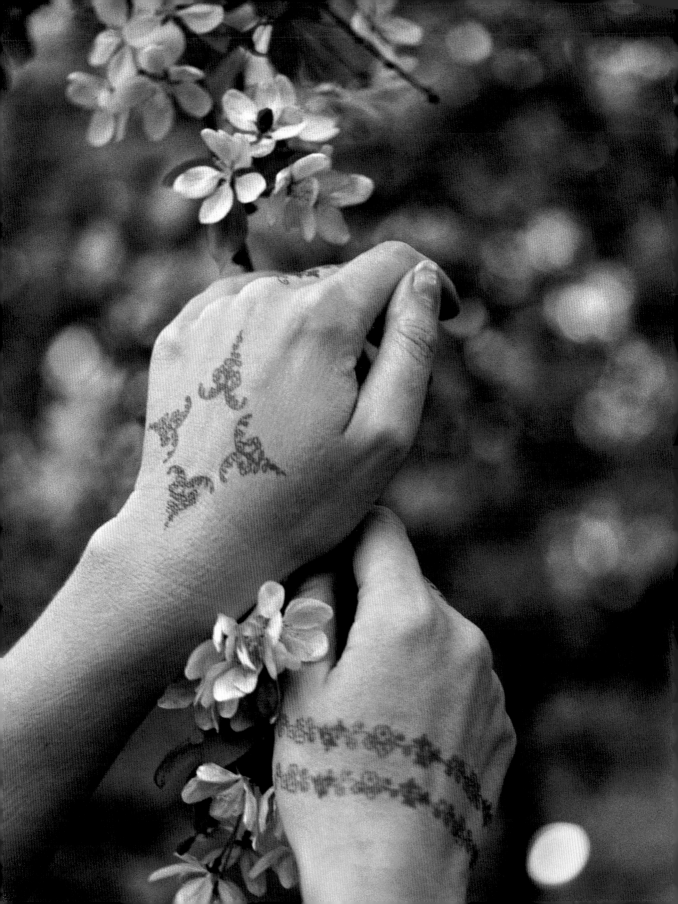

British Beauty Hand Treatment

A friend of mine from London with soft, delicate hands swears this recipe works wonders. Benzoin is a preservative.

2 tablespoons cooked or uncooked oatmeal (or colloidal oatmeal)
Water
1 teaspoon almond meal
A few drops almond oil
A few drops tincture of benzoin (optional)

Combine all the ingredients, adding just enough water to form a thick paste. Apply to your hands, put on a pair of cotton gloves, and leave on overnight.

Hot Tomato Hand Lotion

Tomatoes originated in the Andes. The tomato familiar to the Incas was a small, yellow fruit, transported to Europe by the conquistadores. Eventually the fruit made its way back to North America in the early nineteenth century and it became a favorite of Thomas Jefferson, who was (among other things, of course) an eminent horticulturist. Tomatoes are rich in vitamin C, which is excellent for the skin. Their acidity has exfoliating properties that help to renew the epidermal cells, a big boost for very dry skin.

Juice of 1 overripe tomato
1 teaspoon glycerin
1 teaspoon apple cider vinegar

Whisk all the ingredients together. Apply all over your hands. Leave on for 5 to 10 minutes, then rinse off. Bottle the leftover lotion, label, and refrigerate. Shake well before using. The lotion will keep for a few days in the refrigerator.

MEHNDI

Hands and feet have been used as a canvas for rich ornamentation since prehistoric times: cave art depicts painted and ornamented hands. Mehndi is the traditional art of painting and adorning the hands and feet with red or dark brown powdered henna and other ingredients (some women use eucalyptus oil, tea, sugar, methi seeds, and tamarind paste). While often associated with India, there is some historical evidence that the use of henna to create these intricate designs may have originated in North Africa, worked its way through the Middle East, and arrived on the subcontinent with the Moguls in the twelfth century.

In India, mehndi is an important component of ceremonies and rituals. Upper-caste brides, swathed in silks, jewels, and perfumes, have their hands and feet painted with an intricate tracery of designs. Tradition says that the deeper the color, the longer the couple's love will last. The henna used in mehndi design is thought to have special powers, warding off evil spirits and the evil eye.

Lately, mehndi has come into vogue among Western women. There has been a rash of books published and seminars offered, and, of course, celebrities have been spotted with the delicate patterns on their hands and feet.

Celtic Pride Hand Nourisher

Oatmeal has always been a favorite breakfast treat among my Irish relatives. My aunt told me that Irish women used to cleanse their hands with porridge, oatmeal, or almond meal to keep them soft and smooth.

2 tablespoons oatmeal (or almond meal)
1 to 2 teaspoons almond oil
A few drops apple cider vinegar
1 tablespoon honey

Combine all the ingredients to form a thick paste. Apply all over your hands, and put on a pair of cotton gloves. Leave on for as long as you can or overnight.

La Vie en Rose

Around the tenth century, provincial French-men began the manufacture of rosewater, still a favorite among Frenchwomen. In Islamic tradition, the rose was the most loved and sacred

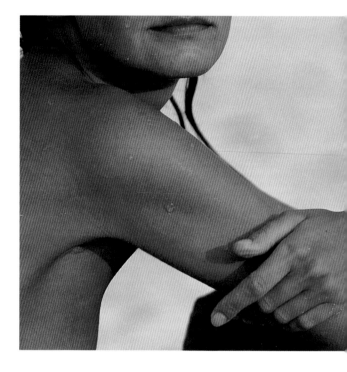

flower, and rosewater was the scent of choice among Arab women.

4 ounces distilled water
1 to 2 drops rose essential oil

To make your own homemade "rosewater" add the rose oil to the distilled water. For a larger batch, add a very small vial of rose oil to 1 gallon of distilled water. You can then put the rosewater in small individual bottles to give as gifts.

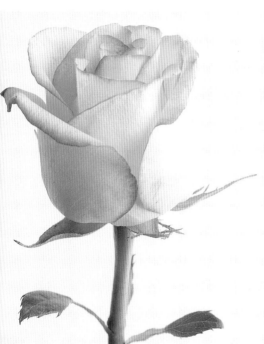

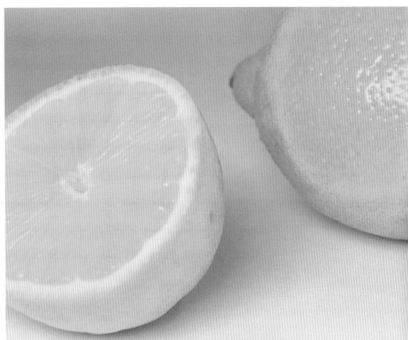

Rosewater Hand Moisturizer

Glycerin and rosewater are ancient remedies. Used for thousands of years in cosmetics, the combination works wonders as a moisturizer and emollient. The rosewater acts as a gentle astringent. This skin cream is wonderful for all skin types, including sensitive skin.

2 to 3 tablespoons glycerin
2 to 3 tablespoons corn starch
1/2 cup rosewater (see La Vie en Rose)

A few drops freshly squeezed lemon juice

In a small saucepan over low heat, combine the glycerin and corn starch. Add the rosewater and lemon juice a few drops at a time, until the mixture thickens into a paste. Place in a jar and label. Apply to your hands as a lotion, or put on a pair of cotton gloves and leave on overnight.

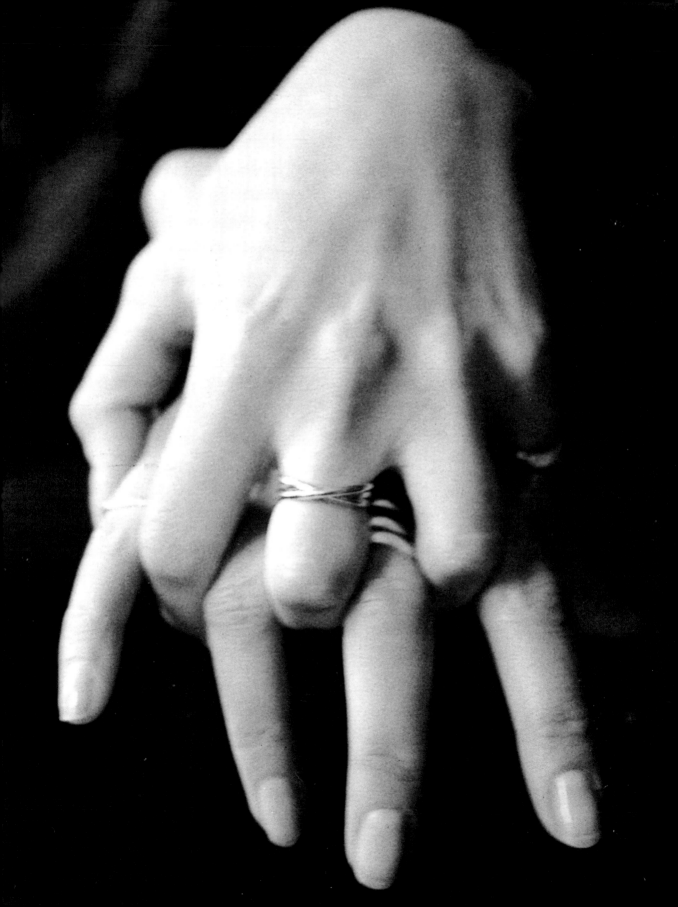

THE HONEY BEE
BRILLIANT AS EINSTEIN'S IDEA
CAN'T BE TAUGHT A THING.
LIKE THE SUN, SHE'S ON COURSE FOREVER.
AS IF NOTHING ELSE AT ALL EXISTED
EXCEPT HER FLOWERS.

TED HUGHES
English, 20th century
from "The Honey Bee"

Quick Rosewater Hand Moisturizer

3 to 4 tablespoons glycerin
1/2 cup rosewater

Combine the ingredients and apply as a lotion, or put the mixture in a shallow dish and soak your hands.

Tahitian Cocoa Butter Hand and Nail Treatment

Made from the oil of the chocolate nut, cocoa butter is a favorite beauty enhancer for skin and hair among the women of Polynesia. I picked up the recipe for this treatment while working in Bora Bora, a tiny island in Tahiti. This is a wonderful skin softener for dry or chapped hands.

4 tablespoons cocoa butter
4 tablespoons almond oil
3 to 4 tablespoons shredded beeswax
5 to 6 tablespoons glycerin (optional)

In a double boiler over low heat, combine the cocoa butter, almond oil, and beeswax, stirring until thoroughly blended and liquefied. Slowly add the glycerin until the mixture is smooth and thick. Place in a jar and label.

Honey Bee Hand Lotion

1 to 2 teaspoons clear honey
3 to 4 tablespoons glycerin
8 to 10 tablespoons rosewater
A few drops apple cider vinegar
or white vinegar

Warm the honey in a saucepan over low heat until it's slightly runny. Remove from the heat and add the remaining ingredients, adding just enough vinegar to make a smooth lotion. Bottle and label. You can wear this lotion to bed at night with a pair of cotton gloves.

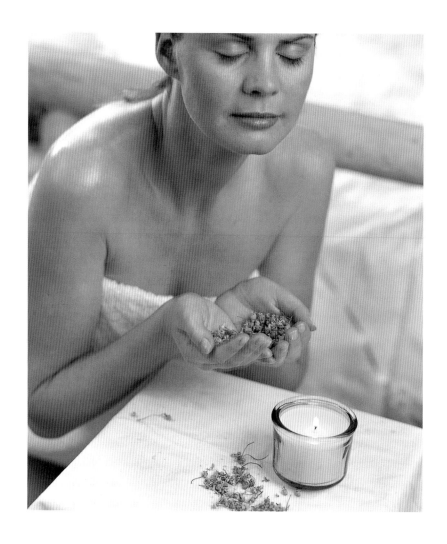

AROMATHERAPY HAND TREATMENTS

Aromatherapy uses the potent essential oils of plants to soothe, stimulate, and heal. There are many theories about how plants use these oils that are found at or near the surface layer of cells. In some plants, they may attract pollinating insects. In others, they may repel harmful fungi. Herbalists have developed ways to harness the varied properties of essential oils, what they refer to as the plant's "life force," for healing.

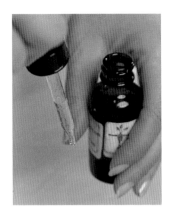 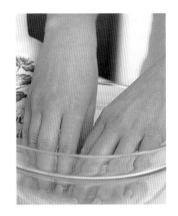 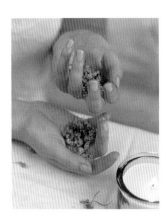

Naturopathica Hand Soak

The following two recipes come from Barbara Close, the owner of Naturopathica Spa in East Hampton, New York. Barbara likes to start her hand treatments with a soak infused with lavender essential oil. She relates that lavender is an antiseptic and will help heal ragged hangnails and prevent nail-bed infections, while its anti-inflammatory properties will calm dermatitis.

2 to 4 drops lavender oil
Water

Fill a bowl large enough to accommodate your fingertips with lukewarm water and add the lavender oil. Soak your hands for 10 minutes.

Naturopathica Cuticle Soother

Barbara likes to follow the previous soak with a cuticle-softening treatment using jojoba oil, rosemary oil, peppermint (to stimulate local circulation in the nail bed), and lavender oil (for its anti-inflammatory properties).

1 tablespoon jojoba oil
4 drops rosemary oil
3 drops peppermint oil
5 drops lavender oil

Combine all the ingredients and massage into your cuticles.

Moonlight in Vermont Moisturizing Lotion

In cold climates during the winter, hands become dry, chapped, and sometimes cracked. Lavender and geranium are soothing to hands and contain skin-healing properties. The delicious scent also serves as reminder that spring is on the way.

1 tablespoon natural, unscented hand lotion
2 drops lavender oil
2 drops geranium oil

Add the essential oils to the lotion. Apply all over your hands and let this sensual lotion absorb into the skin.

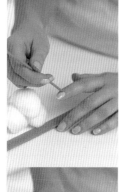

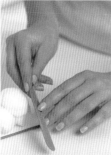

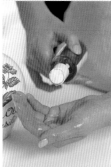

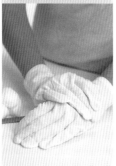

I WAS OBLIGED, AS I GAZED AT HER
TO SUPPRESS THE SMILE THAT IS PROVOKED IN US
BY THE SOLEMNITY, THE INNOCENCE,
AND THE GRACE OF LITTLE CHILDREN.

MARCEL PROUST
French, 19th to 20th century
from *The Captive*

HOME MANICURE

1 The best time to give yourself a manicure is just after a bath or shower. The nails should be clean and soft. Remove all traces of nail polish by moistening a cotton ball or pad with nail polish remover and rubbing from the base of the nail to the tip.

2 Wash your hands in warm water with a mild soap for a few minutes to remove dirt, soften the nails and cuticles, and rinse off the residual nail polish remover.

3 Wrap a cotton ball or pad around each end of an orangewood stick (available at drugstores). Use it to clean under the edge of your nails.

4 Dry your hands on a soft towel, then apply shea butter to moisturize the skin and cuticles.

5 There is some controversy about pushing cuticles back. Dermatologists say that this can damage the cuticle and the surrounding skin, inviting infection. Most beauticians, however, claim that there is no problem if the procedure is done properly. If you do choose to manipulate the cuticle, be extremely gentle and careful. Use an orangewood stick to gently push the cuticles back (in a pinch, use the back of a clean pencil eraser).

6 File the nails with a metal nail file or emery board, using gentle, one-directional strokes—do not use a see-saw motion, as this can cause splitting. Some manicurists suggest holding the file at a 75-degree angle tilting away from the fingertip. This leaves the harder protective top layer of nail cells in place. File the nails into a squared-off oval shape. Avoid filing the sides of the nails, which can cause catching and chipping. Make sure all the nails are the same length.

7 Apply one of the moisturizing creams, oils, or lotions in this book, and massage into your hands and cuticles. Put on a pair of cotton gloves and leave on for at least 30 minutes or overnight, if possible. Your hands will be super-soft and your nails will be well-nourished.

8 Put a small amount of nail cream, vegetable oil, or beeswax on each nail, and buff with a leather buffer for a natural shine. Buffing also increases circulation to the nails.

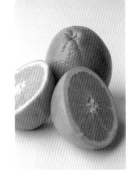

Neroli Hand Cream

This lemon-yellow oil created from orange blossoms was named for Anna Maria de la Tremoille, the Princess of Neroli. A seventeenth-century Italian noblewoman, Anna Maria was obsessed with the scent and set a fashion for perfuming hair, clothing, and baths with orange flowers. Neroli has calming properties and was also very popular with Victorian ladies. This recipe is great for soothing chapped or overworked hands.

1 tablespoon unscented natural hand lotion
1 drop neroli essential oil
1 drop carrot essential oil

Add the essential oils to the lotion. Massage into your hands and nails.

To Deodorize Hands

- Rub freshly cut lemons over your hands.

- Cut a small white potato in half and rub the cut sides over hands.

- Combine equal parts lemon juice and white wine vinegar. Wash your hands with the mixture. It will soften the hands and work as a deodorizer. The vinegar acts as a preservative, so you can bottle and label the leftover mixture and store some for later.

Nail Treatments

Your fingernails protect the sensitive ends of your fingers from trauma and are equally useful as tools for gouging and grasping. The nail is made of a protein called keratin and is actually considered epidermal material, like the skin.

Since hard labor can be so punishing to nails, in many societies around the world, long, perfect nails are considered a symbol of upper-class luxury. However, well-tended nails are no longer the exclusive entitlement of the rich. Basic manicuring is simple, inexpensive, and should be done at least once a week. It is also wise to see a professional manicurist at least every 4 to 6 weeks to keep your nails looking healthy and beautiful.

A proper diet is also essential. Protein deficiencies can make nails brittle, weak, and dull-looking. Eat plenty of vegetable protein, sprouts, leafy greens, whole grains, and seafood. Silicon-rich foods like sea vegetables, onions, broccoli, and fish are also great for your nails.

EVERYDAY HAND TIPS

- Always wear gloves when doing household chores, kitchen cleanups, washing dishes, or working in the yard.
- Keep a bottle of hand cream or lotion by the bathroom and kitchen sinks. Use after each wash.
- Keep a bottle of hand cream or lotion beside your bed and use every night before you go to sleep.

NAIL CARE TIPS

- To treat and prevent peeling, avoid harsh nail polish removers, detergents, chemicals, and dark nail polishes. To speed up recovery, cut your nails short, buff them, then apply vitamin E oil or lotion twice a day. Try not to polish for three to four weeks.

- For brittle nails, massage with castor oil daily for one month.

- For discolored nails, rub fresh lemon juice around the nail base.

- Give nails a break from polish. Allow them to breathe for at least one day a week and for one week every month or so.

- Before polishing, apply some vinegar. It cleans the nails, providing a more even surface for the polish, so it will last longer.

- To strengthen weak nails, soak daily for five minutes in warm olive oil or apple cider vinegar.

- For nails that are stained or dirty, use a Q-tip or orangewood stick with a cotton tip soaked in water mixed with a little bleach, then rub directly on the stain. You can also use an old toothbrush or nail brush with a soap or bleach solution to scrub nails and remove stains.

- To stimulate circulation to your nails, press down for about 10 seconds on the moon (the round part at the bottom) of each nail. Repeat two to three times.

Henna Nail Polish

The ancient Chinese are credited as being the first to polish, or paint, their nails. Henna was used by the ancient Egyptians to dye the fingernails, soles of the feet, and the palms of the hands. In India women paint henna on their hands and feet for special occasions.

1 to 2 teaspoons red henna

Add enough water to the henna to make a thin paste. Paint the henna onto your nails and let dry, preferably in the sun. Rinse off. The nails will look pink, and because it is a stain, there is no chipping. This stain will remain until the new nail grows out.

Antillean Papaya Cuticle Softener

Over the centuries, women from the Caribbean islands have devised clever ways of combating the hot Antillean sun. The active enzymes in papaya and pineapple juice soften cuticles.

2 tablespoons fresh papaya or pineapple juice
2 egg yolks
1/2 teaspoon vinegar or lemon juice

Combine all the ingredients in a small bowl. Soak your nails in the mixture for at least 30 minutes.

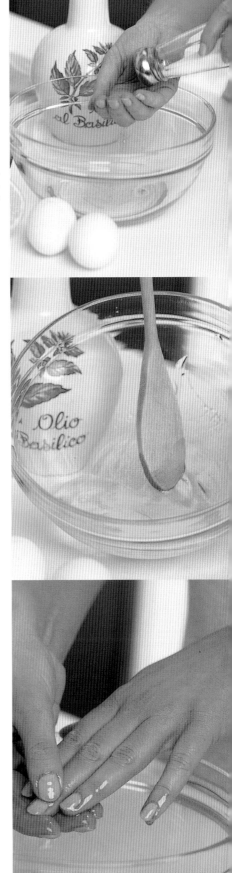

Avocado Oil Nail Restoration "Cream"

Avocados were cultivated by the Aztecs, who believed they had aphrodisiacal powers. The rich flesh of the fruit is about 20 percent oil.

1 teaspoon honey
1 teaspoon avocado oil
1 egg yolk
A few drops apple cider vinegar
A pinch sea salt

Combine all the ingredients and rub the mixture into your nails. Leave on for 30 minutes, then rinse.

Milk Maid Hand and Cuticle Softener

Milk has been used for centuries as a beauty treatment.

1 to 2 cups warm milk or buttermilk

Soak your hands in the milk for 10 to 15 minutes. This will soften and smooth skin and cuticles. Then file the nails gently and push back the cuticles with an orangewood stick.

145

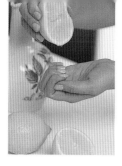

Ladies Who Lunch Nail Whitener

Better than a pair of little white gloves. Olive oil is very effective in treating brittle nails.

1/4 cup olive oil
1/4 cup freshly squeezed lemon juice

Warm the olive oil in a saucepan over low heat. Dip your nails in the oil for 5 to 10 minutes. After dipping, massage each nail individually. Massage your hands using the remaining oil. Gently push back the cuticles with an orangewood stick and shape the nails using an emery board. Blot any excess oil. Rub the nails with the lemon juice to whiten them.

Bora Bora Coconut and Essential Oil Nail Warmer

The heat and coconut oil in this recipe help dry, brittle nails absorb moisture.

3 to 4 ounces coconut oil
5 drops chamomile oil
5 drops lavender oil
5 drops geranium oil
2 drops ylang-ylang oil

Warm the coconut oil in a saucepan over low heat. Add the essential oils. Massage this wonderfully nourishing, aromatic oil into your hands and nails.

Yucatan Jojoba Oil Nail Treatment

While traveling through Mexico, I stayed at a charming resort area called Playa del Carmen in the Yucatan. One of the local women there told me of this nail treatment.

1/4 cup jojoba oil or sweet almond oil
5 drops lemon essential oil

Warm the jojoba oil in a saucepan over low heat, then add the lemon oil. Massage the oil mixture into hands and nails and leave on for a few minutes. Gently push back the cuticles with an orangewood stick and shape the nails using an emery board. Blot any excess oil.

Flaxseed Hand and Nail Soak

Flax has been an important crop in Europe, Africa, and Asia for more than 5,000 years. The production of flax fibers into textiles is one of humankind's oldest manufacturing processes. Varieties of flax are variously made into linen thread, used for animal feed, and used as a base for oil paints.

1/4 cup flaxseed oil
(available at health-food stores)
1/4 cup olive oil
A few drops tincture of benzoin

In a bowl large enough for both your hands, combine the oils. If you like, you might want to warm the oils slightly. Soak your hands in the oils for about 10 minutes, then rinse with water and tincture of benzoin. Your hands will feel nourished and smooth.

DOWN BY THE SALLEY GARDENS MY LOVE AND I DID MEET:
SHE PASSED THE SALLEY GARDENS WITH LITTLE SNOW-WHITE FEET.

WILLIAM BUTLER YEATS
Irish, 19th to 20th century
from "Down by the Salley Gardens"

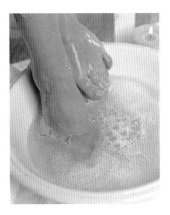

FEET

Aside from their more pedestrian functions, feet are often the object of amorous attention and heightened sexuality. Regency bucks admired a shapely ankle. Victorians swooned over a glimpse of dainty, childlike feet. High heels are associated with kept women in many cultures. Geishas set the fashion in Japan for high-platformed sandals to keep their feet above the mud of the street, and French courtesans experimented with high heels as a way of elongating and emphasizing the legs and feet.

These women paid a price for fashion, as does the modern lady teetering about in the latest vertiginous-heeled shoe. But even so-called sensible shoes can do a number on feet that are standing or walking all day. Tired, sore feet can affect your overall person; if you treat your feet badly, your whole body feels miserable. A foot soak or a self-massage for the feet will revitalize you, dissolve your stress, and relax you.

Foot Soaks

Foot soaks are wonderful for relieving fatigued, aching feet after a stressful or active day. A good foot soak will open the pores and draw toxins out of the system, and a few drops of scented essential oil added to your warm foot bath can restore a sense of well-being to your entire body.

Not surprisingly, societies known for their sensual extravagances were the earliest to use foot baths for medicinal as well as pleasurable purposes. The Romans, for example, were big on bathing the feet; they appreciated the therapeutic value of immersing feet in warm, healing springs. In the nineteenth century, French spas prescribed foot baths to soothe arthritis. A little natural powder (talc) after your foot bath will help you put on your shoes, especially in hot weather.

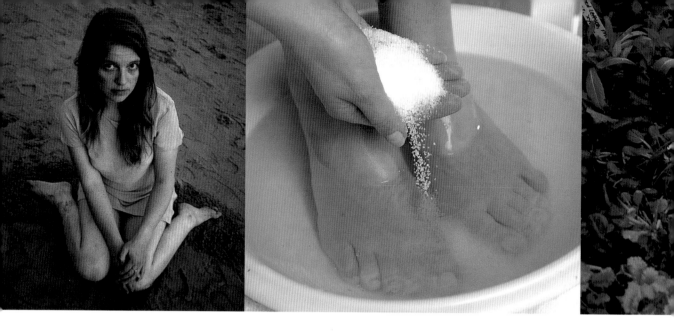

Seashore Soak

Salt has powerful healing properties. You can use regular salt, but I prefer sea salt. The salt water will remind you of wading in the surf on sunny beaches.

2 tablespoons sea salt

Add the salt to two pints of warm water. Soak your feet for 10 to 20 minutes.

Epsom Salt Soak

Epsom salts are minerals that have cathartic properties and have been used in baths for aching feet and sore bodies.

2 tablespoons Epsom salts

Add the Epsom salts to three quarts of warm water. Soak your feet for 10 to 20 minutes.

Father Kneipp's Hot and Cold Foot Bath

Father Kneipp was a pioneer in the benefits and therapeutic uses of water and foot baths. Alternating the feet between tubs of hot and cold water can relieve foot fatigue and is wonderfully invigorating and energizing. Fill two tubs, one with very warm to hot water and the second with cold. The water in each tub should be at least 8 inches deep. Place your feet first in the hot tub for about 3 minutes, then switch to the cold water for 30 to 40 seconds. Repeat the procedure twice, always ending with the cold water.

Aromatherapy Foot Baths

To create an aromatherapy foot bath, start with a good foot basin (you can find a purpose-made one in drug or medical supply stores) or tub large enough to accommodate both feet up to at least ankle level. You can add essential oils to unscented bath gels or bath salts. Make sure the water is warm, not too hot,

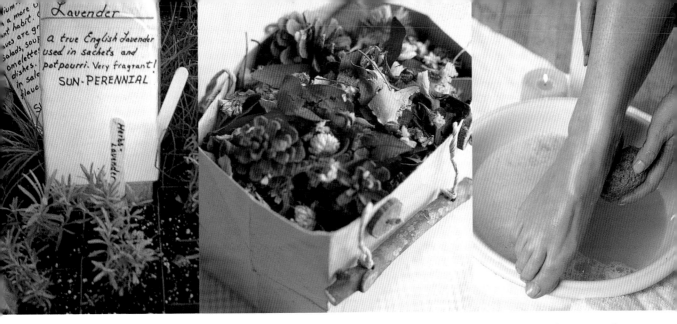

when adding essential oils; otherwise, the oils will evaporate too quickly.

For a quick, all-purpose foot bath, add 8 to 10 drops of essential oil, or a combination of oils, to 1 to 2 cups of Epsom salts or sea salt and warm water. Alternatively, add 10 to 15 drops of essential oil or oils to one ounce of unscented bath gel.

Experiment with different combinations: add 5 to 10 drops of essential oils or an essential oil blend (mixed with a carrier oil, like olive or almond) to 3 quarts of water. Gently stir the oils around with your hand to disperse the oil before soaking your feet.

Lavender Foot Soak

Lavender oil contains properties that help relieve fatigue and was also used to clean sick rooms in ancient Greece, Rome, and Persia. Its name comes from the Latin, meaning "to clean."

5 to 10 drops lavender oil

Add the oil to 2 to 3 quarts of warm water. Soak your feet for 10 to 20 minutes.

Always consult an aromatherapy manual before custom blending or selecting essential oils. Many are very potent and should not be used if you have medical conditions like high blood pressure, epilepsy, or are pregnant. It is always wise to consult your physician if you have any questions. Because of their intensity, some essential oils do not require as many drops to achieve the desired strength.

Walkabout Tea Tree Foot Bath

The aboriginal peoples of Australia use tea tree essential oil for its antiseptic properties. Lavender also has antiseptic and soothing properties.

2 drops tea tree oil
2 drops lavender oil

Add the essential oils to a tub of warm water. Soak your feet for 10 minutes. It is wonderfully relaxing.

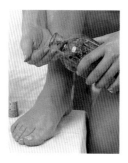 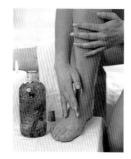

Massage

Foot massage is wonderful for releasing stress. Stroking, kneading, and rubbing the feet awakens the rest of your body. In the evening or after a bath, try rubbing your feet with a light, vegetable-based oil (sesame oil is nice) or an unscented lotion, with a few drops of essential oils added. Then rest with a few pillows tucked under your feet.

Better yet, for a deliciously sensual experience, ask your partner to massage your feet. A Roman visitor to Cleopatra's court noted that Mark Antony rubbed her feet at dinner, taking it as a sign of his countryman's subservience to the Egyptian queen. For a more enlightened observer, it might rather have been a sign of Antony's devotion. A man once told me that every night for the past 25 years he has given his wife a foot massage; he swears it keeps his marriage going.

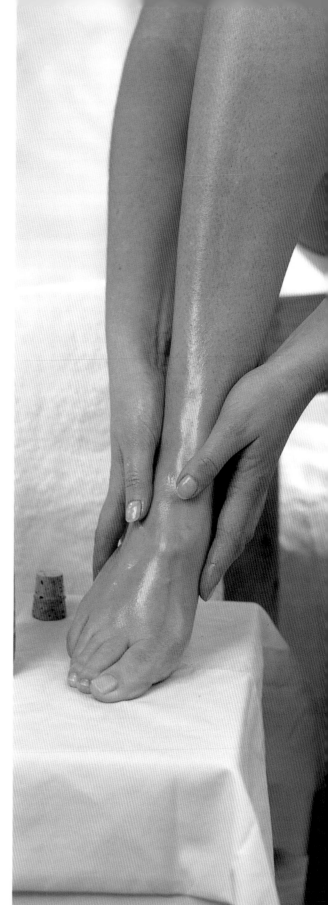

THEN TOOK MARY A POUND OF OINTMENT OF SPIKENARD, VERY COSTLY,
AND ANOINTED THE FEET OF JESUS, AND WIPED HIS FEET WITH HER HAIR;
AND THE HOUSE WAS FILLED WITH THE ODOUR OF THE OINTMENT.

JOHN 12:3
1st century A.D.
The Bible

Foot massage is a symbol of respect and devotion in many spiritual texts. Massaging with nourishing oils and essential oils will improve circulation, soften the skin, and help slough off dry skin. It is of course also a wonderful way to relax and pamper yourself. Start out with a nourishing base oil; you can try any one or a combination of sesame oil, grapeseed oil, sweet almond, jojoba, or safflower oils. To custom blend your own, add a few drops of essential oil. A good rule of thumb is to add 10 to 15 drops of essential oil per 2 tablespoons of base oil.

Balinese Secret for Aching Feet

The resorts and spas of Bali are famous for their pampering. Balinese therapists often use clove foot oils and foot scrubs. Clove oil is an antiseptic and can act as a temporary, local anesthetic. Use clove oil sparingly since it is very strong and can be irritating to some skin types. If you have sensitive skin, test this oil on a small area first.

5 tablespoons sesame oil
4 drops clove essential oil

Combine the ingredients, then gently massage the oil into your feet. Bottle the remainder and label.

Peppermint Sports Foot Oil

This is a great blend for after your workout. The combination of peppermint, orange, and tea tree essential oils are a great pick-me-up for tired feet. Many people find tea tree oil effective against athlete's foot. The grapeseed oil acts as a preservative.

2 teaspoons sweet almond oil
3 teaspoons grapeseed oil
2 drops peppermint oil
2 drops orange oil
1 drop tea tree oil

Combine all the ingredients, then gently massage into your feet. This recipe makes enough for a single foot massage, but you can always make more if you like, then bottle and label.

HEAVEN, I'M IN HEAVEN,
AND MY HEART BEATS SO THAT
I CAN HARDLY SPEAK,
AND I SEEM TO FIND THE HAPPINESS I SEEK
WHEN WE'RE OUT TOGETHER
DANCING CHEEK TO CHEEK.

IRVING BERLIN
American, 20th century
from "Cheek to Cheek"

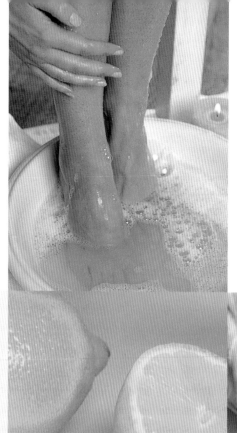

Sweet Citrus Smoother Scrub

Calendula, or pot marigold, is a favorite medicinal herb whose petals were applied to wounds by Civil War nurses to stanch the flow of blood. It can also be used for everything from soothing rashes to treating toothaches. This concoction smells deliciously citrusy and is a great escape if you can't make it to the beach.

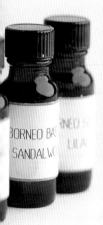

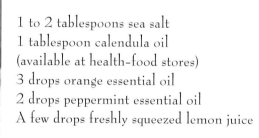

1 to 2 tablespoons sea salt
1 tablespoon calendula oil
(available at health-food stores)
3 drops orange essential oil
2 drops peppermint essential oil
A few drops freshly squeezed lemon juice

In a small bowl, combine the salt with the oils and lemon juice until the salt is evenly moistened. Soak your feet in a foot bath (see the recipes in this chapter) to soften the skin, then pat your feet dry with a towel. Massage the scrub into your feet for 5 minutes, paying special attention to rough and callused areas. Rinse with warm water and pat dry. If you like, put on warm cotton socks to continue softening the feet.

REFLEXOLOGY

Reflexology is a method of manipulation of the feet (and hands) that can help a wide variety of conditions, from asthma to arthritis. The basic premise of reflexology is that there are specific areas or points on the feet and hands that are connected to all other parts of the body—including the organs, glands, nerves, and muscles. Pressure from stress and strain can irritate nerve endings in the feet, which in turn can cause problems in the corresponding parts of the body. Rubbing, twisting, or kneading these points in the feet causes a "reflex" effect, releasing pressure in the feet and sending energy elsewhere in the body. For instance, working on the toes is meant to soothe pain in the head and neck; loosening up the ankle is said to improve problems in the pelvic region.

THE BARE NECESSITIES

I love the feeling of walking around without shoes or socks. When summer comes, I dispense with them whenever possible. Long, barefoot walks on the beach are wonderful for your feet and legs, and the sand provides a terrific foot massage. The sand also acts as a natural pumice and helps wear down calluses and rough skin. After a long walk in the sand my calves always feel strengthened. Walking barefoot in the grass can also be soothing and a wonderful way to connect with the earth.

Try some simple foot exercises to increase circulation and help eliminate toxins. You can do these exercises almost anywhere, and they're especially good at helping diffuse tension in stressful situations—on a plane, in a classroom, during a meeting (under the conference table, of course).

Flex and rotate your feet and ankles whenever possible. Stretch your whole body and toes the minute you get out of bed; sit on your heels and stretch your toes. Japanese women often do this exercise, as it helps develop good posture and improves blood circulation throughout the body.

Summer Feet Sweet Relief

This is a wonderfully cooling treat for hot, sticky, aching feet.

2 teaspoons apple cider vinegar

Wash or soak your feet in warm water, then splash with cool water and pat dry with a towel. Pour the apple cider vinegar into the palms of your hands and massage into the feet, especially the soles. Sweet relief!

HOME PEDICURE

1. Add 1 to 2 tablespoons of almond oil or a mild soap to about 3 quarts of warm water. Soak your feet for about 10 to 15 minutes to soften the skin. While soaking, gently massage away any calluses or hard skin with a pumice stone. Be sure to keep your feet and the pumice stone wet. When your feet are smooth, pat them dry with a towel.

2. Cut the toenails. Always cut straight across to prevent ingrown toenails, then use an emery board to smooth out sharp or rough edges.

3. Use an orangewood stick to gently push back cuticles. I like to soften my cuticles with jojoba oil or almond oil first.

4. Use a leather buffer to buff the nails to a shine (buffing also increases circulation).

5. Apply a soothing lotion and gently massage your feet. Your feet should look and feel beautiful.

I WALK TO FIND YOU
SOMETIMES FIVE OR SIX MILES—
CHERRIES IN BLOSSOM

BASHO
Japanese, 17th century

Chapter Five

BEAUTY IN BALANCE

The quest for beauty is a profoundly human urge. We seek it in the world around us, we strive to cultivate it in ourselves, we long to fill our lives with it. Although different cultures and different eras may define exactly what is beautiful in various ways, the poet's yearning for the exquisite scent and sight and sensation of spring blossoms is something every sentient being can know.

Clearly our appreciation of beauty goes beyond the pleasurable reaction to a pretty face. Likewise, feeling beautiful is more than painting on full lips or liposuctioning away unwanted curves. It seems a bit of an old chestnut, but the saying is true: Beauty comes from inside. When mind, body, and spirit are in balance, you are well on your way to genuine, lasting beauty. Beauty comes from a mind and body in sync with each other—and with the natural world.

Perhaps it is not so surprising, then, that in an era filled with the promises of high technology and modern medicine, we are reaching back to the wisdom of traditional cultures

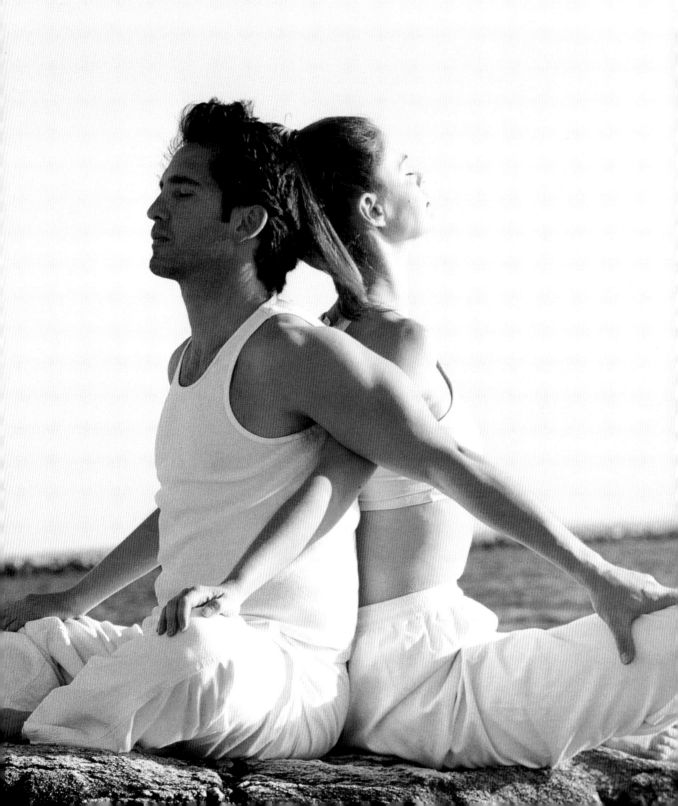

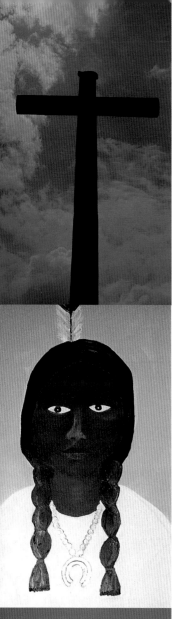

and indigenous peoples to find our true beauty, cure our ills, and ease our minds. Ancient philosophies focus on a holistic, interconnected approach: promoting long-term good health, rather than triaging illness; ministering to the whole person, not just the specific problem. Slowly but surely, the medical establishment is beginning to acknowledge the vital concept of balancing a healthy mind and spirit with a healthy body.

The ability to discover and draw from inner resources of health, strength, and tranquility is essential to achieving an individual, balanced beauty that radiates from the inside. Yet in a culture dominated by unrealistic ideals of physical beauty, it has become increasingly difficult—but more important than ever—to discover within ourselves that which truly defines beauty: clarity of mind, sense of purpose, physical well-being, and spiritual fulfillment.

The Native American symbol for medicine is a large circle, a hoop that represents the interconnectedness of all things: man and nature, mind and body, living and nonliving, faith and healing. This chapter brings together and expands upon points raised in previous chapters, demonstrating how things like proper diet, exercise, relaxation, and a connection with the natural world are the keys to true beauty.

On the spiritual side are some suggestions about relaxation, meditation, and healing; these techniques are also capable of having positive physiological effects—strengthening bones, limbering muscles, expanding cardiopulmonary capacity. On the physical side are a few basic ideas about fitness and nutrition—a plan that can also help improve mental acuity, combat depression, and promote emotional well-being. Simply, what's good for the body is good for the mind, and vice versa.

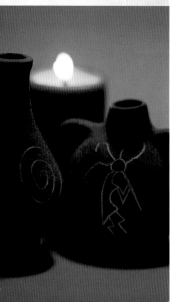

In many parts of the world, philosophies have developed over the millennia that blur the distinction between physical and mental activity. Originally the province of priests, taught by masters to acolytes in ashrams and lamasaries, these activities quickly spread throughout entire populations, and came to be practiced daily by people from all walks of life.

In the nineteenth century, Europe and America went through a phase of spiritualism and "discovered" some of these Eastern disciplines. With the advent of the twentieth century and the passion for things modern and mechanized, the fascination with things like yoga and mysticism went out of fashion, only to resurface in the '60s as people dissatisfied with conventional belief systems looked farther afield for enlightenment.

These disciplines can be especially useful to older people and those with disabilities or who are recovering from an illness, but anyone can benefit from the slow, gentle exercises and the positive effect they have on hormonal balance, alleviating depression, and increasing strength and flexibility.

One of the important differences between these activities and a typical workout exercise is the emphasis on process. While many exercise programs exhort you to push and strain, to change what's "wrong" with your body, these disciplines focus on developing awareness of the body as it is, accepting and working within its limits.

Aside from the benefits of a mentally and physically integrated approach to wellness, yoga and tai chi are particularly effective because their fundamental teachings can be applied to all aspects of life. Thus, unlike setting aside an hour, separate and distinct from the rest of the day, to exercise, these techniques can become a way of life—an integral part of a better, more balanced life.

Yoga

Yoga, developed in India at least three thousand years ago, is a discipline of breath control, meditation, and physical exercise that promotes mental and physical well-being. The word "yoga" is a Sanskrit word meaning "union, concentration, yoking." It follows then that the purpose of the philosophy and technique is to achieve a heightened moment-to-moment awareness, and, ultimately, to attain spiritual enlightenment.

The principles of yoga are an integral part of the *Bhagavad Gita*, "the Song of God," a section of the *Mahabharata* and one of the primary Indian religious texts outlining the ways to achieve *moksha*, meaning "liberation." The *Yoga-sustras*, written by Patanjali in the first century B.C., is something of a training manual of yogic practices and defines yoga as "that which stills the mind."

There are many different types of yoga— bhakti, jnana, karma, kundalini, laya, raja. One of the most popular forms in the West is hatha yoga, which stresses strengthening, toning, and relaxation. Most yoga exercises focus on proper positioning of the body in various *asanas*, or postures, to strengthen and align the spinal column, thought to be the location of the *chakras*, or the body's centers of energy. Yoga improves strength, suppleness, and circulation; promotes relaxation; and increases range of motion, thereby reducing the likelihood of muscle strain (Bletcher, 52).

Yogis believe that breath is the bridge between the mind and body. *Pranayama* are specific exercises in which the practitioner breathes deeply, concentrating on the breath as it enters and exits the nostrils. This focus on breathing allows deep muscle relaxation, releases tension, and induces a tranquil state.

Slowly, gently expanding the entire area of the lungs reproduces the way the body operates during sleep or meditation. It's a signal that the body is in a relaxed state. Conversely, shallow chest breathing triggers the nervous system's "fight-or-flight" mechanism; it replicates a state of high stress. Short, through-the-mouth breaths put the body in a state of readiness for quick, decisive action. In this condition, the body reacts as if it is in an emergency state and produces stress-induced chemicals like adrenaline.

Yoga breathing techniques have been used by professional athletes to improve performance. By breathing deeply through the nose, oxygen is drawn into the lower lungs. The lower lungs contain more blood and have greater oxygen-exchange capacity. Therefore, oxygen, essential for muscle function, can be delivered in higher concentrations to fuel the muscles.

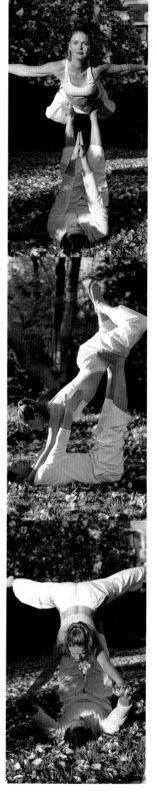

Benefits of Yoga

Yoga has been shown to:

- *lower blood pressure*
- *increase energy*
- *relieve stress and mild depression*
- *increase balance, strength, and flexibility*
- *improve concentration and memory*
- *induce a sense of calmness*
- *improve hormonal function*

(Harvard Health Letter)

ON-THE-JOB STRESS SOOTHERS

When Christie Brinkley needs a little R&R, she turns to Dr. Joe Caraccilo, a chiropracter and yoga instructor in New York City, whose high-flying clientele come to him for a little down time. Here are his suggestions for how to combat tension and fatigue when you are on the job. These exercises are quick and easy and can be done virtually anywhere, any time you need a break. An instructor can help you with the postures and be sure you are doing them correctly. The images on the left illustrate a type of contact yoga with Dr. Caraccilo.

Life at work can be very stressful. To still the restlessness of the mind without leaving your work area can be a valuable tool, turning a hectic morning into a serene afternoon. Before you get into the *asanas*, calm the mind with a simple breathing exercise. Breathing is an integral aspect of yoga. It generates heat (to soften muscles), relaxes the body, and helps block out distractions. Deep breathing expands the stomach during inhalation, which drops the diaphragm down and creates a vacuum that can draw more air into the lungs.

1. Place your hand on your stomach; take a deep breath through your nose and feel your stomach expand like a balloon.

2. Exhale through your nose while pulling your stomach inward. This forcefully expels the air, making more room for the next breath.

3. Repeat 15 to 20 times. Now you are ready to do the posture work.

THE ASANAS

1. *The Eagle Posture Variation.* This position relaxes the neck and shoulders while opening the chest. Sitting up straight in your chair, open your arms out to each side as though you were preparing to hug someone. Now bring your arms inward as if to hug yourself, interlace your forearms, crossing one elbow over the other, and bring your palms together in a prayer position. Lift your elbows toward the ceiling and tilt your head back to get the full stretch.

2. *The Seated Spinal Twist.* If you sit in your chair all morning, the muscles of your back will inevitably tighten up. This asana will help alleviate pressure in the mid and lower back, promoting relaxation and allowing the creative energy to flow. Sitting straight in your chair, rotate your upper body to the right, grasping the far end of the back of your chair with your right hand and the near end of the chair with your left. Get a good grip and rotate your torso to the right looking over your right shoulder. Take 5 deep breaths and repeat on to the left side.

3. *The Tree Posture.* When things seem to be getting out of hand around the office and a little grounding is called for, this is the remedy. In this asana the standing leg represents the root and trunk of a tree, providing stability and strength, while the arms are the branches free to sway in the wind. Take off your shoes. Standing on your left leg, raise the right foot and place the sole on the left inner thigh (hang in there) with knee out to the side, holding on to the back of a chair to steady yourself. Slowly bring your palms together at the chest in a prayer position. Take 5 breaths and repeat with the opposite leg.

Tai Chi and Qi Gong

Walk the streets of Beijing in the early morning and you'll see groups of people engaged in what looks like an exotic, slow-moving dance. In the park at sunset, perhaps an older gentleman will be going through the motions under a favorite tree. These exercises are interconnected with a vast socioreligious system that encompasses endemic cultural values like discipline, respect for nature, and inner strength and balance.

Tai chi and qi gong are widely practiced throughout China. Factory workers take a tai chi break during the day to calm the spirit, clear the mind, and return to work relaxed and more productive. The series of graceful exercises is based on the motions of the natural world and emphasizes groundedness, fluidity, and balance. Sped up, the strength and purpose of these movements can be used in self-defense, as one of the martial arts.

Qi gong (pronounced "chi gung") is an ancient Chinese healing technique dating back more than three thousand years. This form of "meditation in motion" involves stretching, rhythmic breathing, mental concentration, and circular, flowing movements thought to change the flow of energy inside and outside the body. More active forms of qi gong combine dancelike movements with yoga.

Tai chi is a descendant of qi gong. Often described as an internal martial art, tai chi focuses on controlling the body's energy flow through slow, fluid motions requiring intense control and the smooth transfer of weight and movement from one part of the body to another. The movements, also based on forces of nature, are performed to harmonize the circulation of chi, or "life force," in and around the body, and to open up the body to allow chi from the universe to enter.

Both qi gong and tai chi promote deep relaxation, reduce stress, and enhance focus, strength, and balance. Practicing them over time can strengthen the immune system, improve circulation, and even slow the aging process (Colino, 44).

Mental Awareness, Spiritual Healing

Virtually all religious traditions contain a component of meditation. Whether the practitioner concentrates attention on a divine vision, a sacred scripture, a mantra, or his or her own breathing, the purpose of meditation is to empty the mind of extraneous thought. This intensifies focus on the object of contemplation so that the meditator can achieve a greater level of awareness or awakening.

Visualization and guided imagery are meditation techniques that have been adopted and adapted by psychologists and psychotherapists, holistic healers, and sports-medicine practitioners for easing illness, alleviating pain, overcoming stress, anxiety, and depression, and increasing physical and mental performance.

The purpose of all meditation is to concentrate awareness in the present moment, freeing the mind of past regrets or future concerns. It awakens the mind and body, bringing the entire being back into balance.

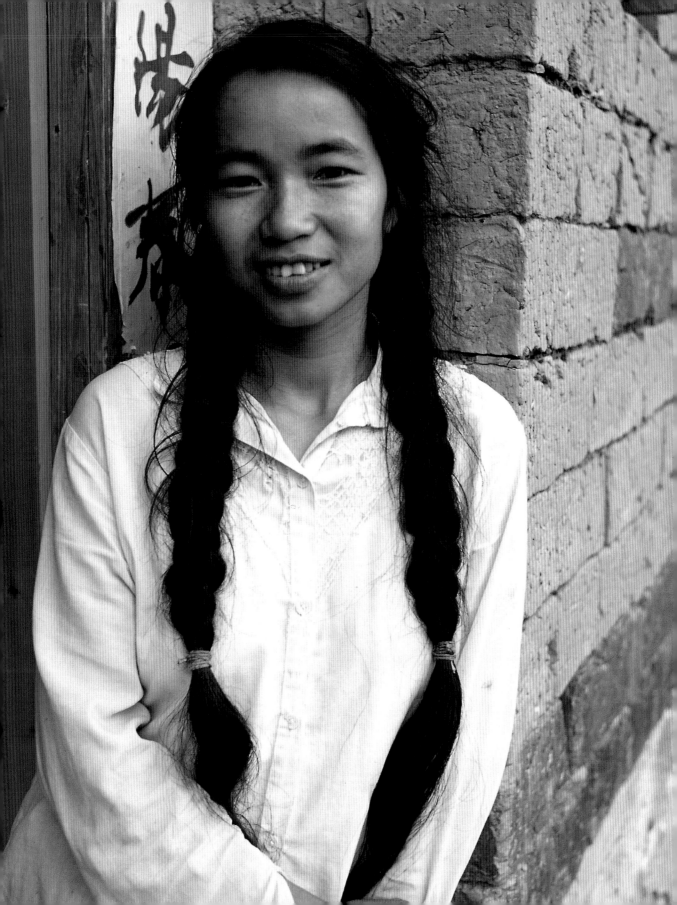

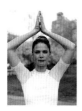
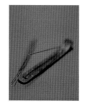
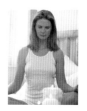

WHEN YOU SAY SOMETHING LIKE "I LOVE YOU" WITH YOUR WHOLE BEING,
NOT JUST WITH YOUR MOUTH OR YOUR INTELLECT, IT CAN TRANSFORM THE WORLD.
A STATEMENT THAT HAS SUCH POWER OF TRANSFORMATION IS CALLED A MANTRA.

THICH NHAT HANH
Vietnamese, 20th century
from *Peace is Every Step*

MEDITATION

Some of the most systematic and effective forms of meditation were developed as part of Buddhist practices. This gentle form of self-healing draws from the Buddhist traditions of compassion for suffering and the search for enlightenment. It was developed to serve rural populations where advanced medical facilities did not exist, so self-help was essential to well-being. Meditation can be done anywhere, anytime, by anyone; it is free, easy, harmless, and has no adverse side effects.

Meditation is a simple technique of heightened self-awareness that induces relaxation, calms the mind, destresses the entire body, and improves physical well-being. Meditation can help break the vicious cycle of stress, worry, fear, and anger that may trigger illness, and then can become the emotional response to illness. Studies have shown that meditation can help you live longer and can alleviate the symptoms of everything from high blood pressure and high cholesterol to drug addiction, depression, cancer, AIDS, and infertility (Kent, 194).

The various forms of meditation described here (from Harp and Feldman, 149) only begin to touch upon the possibilities. Different individuals, like different cultures, can develop their own systems of contemplative being that best suit their needs. You might try one or two techniques for several weeks, then add another, and drop any one that seems less effective. It's not necessary to work exclusively with one type unless you find that this is best for you.

Vipassana or mindfulness meditation. This basic form of meditation promotes heightened self-awareness through contemplating one's breathing and physical sensations in the present moment.

Sit erect, yet relaxed, in a chair or on a cushion on the floor, and concentrate on your breath as it moves in and out of your nostrils. Then focus on each part of your body starting from your toes and working up to your scalp.

Take note of any physical tension you find, as well as any anxieties, fears, or cravings. Don't try to suppress any pain or negative thoughts; rather, acknowledge them, and try to visualize releasing them through your breath. If your mind wanders, bring yourself gently back to the moment by returning to concentrating on the breath.

WALKING MEDITATION

Standing erect,
yet relaxed, walk slowly
back and forth
the length of the room—
or better yet, walk outdoors
across the backyard,
along a beach, or in any
tranquil place.
In addition to concentrating
on your breath as it moves
in and out of your nostrils,
focus on the movements
of your feet as they lift off
the ground, stride forward,
and return to the earth.

TRANSCENDENTAL MEDITATION

This technique involves
the invocation of a mantra,
syllable, word,
or phrase, repeated either
silently or aloud for
several minutes.
This frees the mind from its
continuous internal
dialogue that
subconsciously creates
tension in the body.

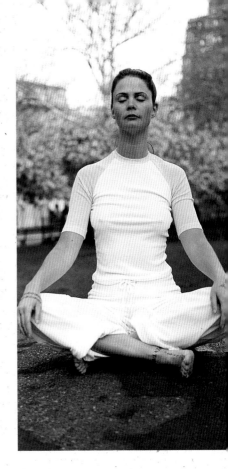

BREATH-COUNTING MEDITATION

Seated comfortably,
breathe deeply in and
out through your
nostrils. Count silently
to yourself,
one number with each
exhalation. If you lose count,
simply start over.
Concentrate on
the breath moving in and
out of your nostrils.

BREATHS-PER-TASK MEDITATION

After practicing
with breath counting,
try this exercise.
Count the number
of breaths it takes
to do a particular
task, for example,
making tea,
folding laundry,
or washing dishes.

FLAME MEDITATION

Light a candle in a
darkened room and stare at
the flame for several
minutes. Try not to think
about anything but the flame
itself. After a few minutes,
blow out the candle,
close your eyes,
and continue to watch
the image of the flame
for as long as it appears.
The more you practice,
the longer you
should be able to
visualize the flame.

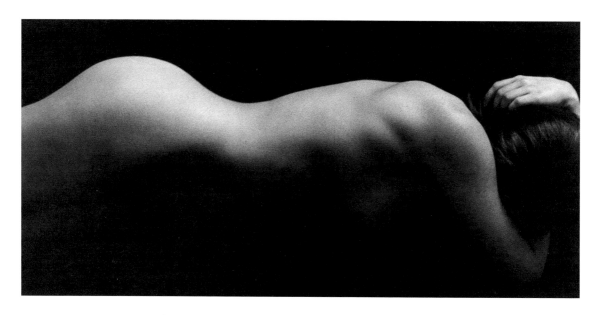

ALL WE ARE IS THE RESULT OF WHAT WE THOUGHT.

SIDDHARTHA GAUTAMA (BUDDHA)

Indian, 6th century B.C.

TIPS FOR EFFECTIVE MEDITATION

- Create a private space where you won't be interrupted; lock the door, unplug the phone, or do whatever it takes to remain uninterrupted and undistracted. If possible, find a quiet place outside.

- Create a soothing atmosphere by playing soft music, lighting a candle, or burning incense. Avoid playing familiar music with lyrics you know by heart, as this can be distracting. Try classical or new-age music, or music from another culture that takes you out of yourself.

- Don't try to meditate on a full or empty stomach. A full stomach uses too much of the body's energy digesting and may cause drowsiness. An empty stomach prevents you from concentrating on anything but food and may cause the body to feel weak.

- If you feel restless or unable to concentrate while sitting still, try a walking meditation or another form of movement meditation such as yoga or tai chi. If you get bored with a mantra, try visualization.

- Be patient. Don't be discouraged if you find it difficult to keep your mind focused. The exercise of constantly returning back to your focal point is part of the process.   *(from Kent, 107)*

THE GREATEST DISCOVERY OF ANY GENERATION IS THAT HUMAN BEINGS
CAN ALTER THEIR LIVES BY ALTERING THEIR ATTITUDES OF MIND.

ALBERT SCHWEITZER

German, 19th to 20th century

Visualization

We are constantly barraged with images from every imaginable form of media. It is therefore not surprising that many people have lost touch with the power of vision and imagination. Many indigenous cultures believe that images held in the mind's eye shape our experience of reality, and they have developed methods to sharpen and manipulate those images. They feel this puts man in greater control of his destiny.

Visualization is a highly effective form of meditation that involves concentrating on images and tapping into the power of the imagination to produce physiological responses. Although we all have daydreams and visions, few of us have learned to take advantage of our imagination in ways that will positively affect our mind and body. Visualization has been used to treat everything from tension headaches to life-threatening diseases.

Visualization and guided imagery are based on the connection between the brain's centers of vision and the autonomic (involuntary) nervous system—the visual cortex of the brain is said to have the ability to influence physical and emotional states. It's akin to the concept of subliminal advertising. The unconscious mind is affected by images the conscious mind can't see.

Images in the mind's eye can shape our experience, so learning to sharpen them can put us more in control of our destiny. If images the brain receives are stress-provoking or unpleasant, the physiological response is negative, unhealthy; if the mental images are pleasant, soothing, and positive, the autonomic nervous system triggers the body's own healing process, enlisting the nervous, endocrine, and immune systems.

Visualization produces greater results if practiced for a few minutes every day, rather than for longer periods less frequently. A few minutes each morning are more productive than an hour once a week. Visualization can be particularly effective if done just before falling asleep or just after waking up, when the body is in a relaxed, transitional state of consciousness. Many people find it helpful to use books or tapes, or simply to recall past moments of great happiness, security, and contentment.

Close your eyes, breathe deeply, and let your mind relive a happy, tranquil moment. Imagine a scene that makes you feel alive, healthy, and relaxed. Revisit times when you have felt confident, strong, and invincible. By concentrating on truly reliving the emotional experience, the mind feeds itself positive images so that the body can recapture the same physical experience and put itself in the same physical state.

Guided Imagery

Like visualization, guided imagery is a simple, effective way of accessing the connection between mind and body. It is sometimes used by the medical community to treat pain and illness. To do this, a trained therapist leads patients into a deeply relaxed state through spoken suggestion and asks them to envision themselves in tranquil surroundings. Patients describe what they see, hear, smell, and feel, in order to reach a deeper state of relaxation. They are asked to visualize their immune system as a strong disease-fighting force. It is believed that cancer patients can heighten immune activity by imagining cancer cells being destroyed by the immune system.

Both guided imagery and visualization are used by professional athletes to improve performance and to overcome the tendency to tense up under pressure.

THE COMBINED ESSENCES OF HEAVEN AND EARTH BECOME THE YIN AND YANG,
THE CONCENTRATED ESSENCES OF THE YIN AND YANG BECOME THE FOUR SEASONS, AND THE
SCATTERED ESSENCES OF THE FOUR SEASONS BECOME THE MYRIAD CREATURES OF THE WORLD.

LIU AN

Chinese, 2nd century B.C.
from *Huai-nan Tzu*

HOLISTIC HEALING

For thousands of years, priests and shamans, nurses and herbalists have practiced naturopathic healing methods. In China, five thousand years ago, the great emperor Fu Hsi laid the groundwork for a system of medicine based on balancing the elements of yin and yang. Twenty-five hundred years later, Taoist medicine was propagated by monks who sought an ideal life of moderation and calm, using a variety of methods to maintain the body's balance.

In ancient Greece, medicine practiced by priests combined diet, meditation, exercise, and herbal remedies. Hippocrates, who promoted the use of scientific methods, was a great proponent of the healing power of nature.

Perhaps the most ancient system of holistic medicine is Ayurveda, whose principles appear in the Vedic scriptures, portions of which date back ten thousand years. Ayurveda comes from the Sanskrit word meaning "the science of prolonging life." The purpose of Ayurveda is to keep the body in balance. It views disease as a lack of balance in the body and approaches treatment as a method of restoring balance.

According to Ayurvedic philosophy, everything a person eats, thinks, and experiences has an impact, positive or negative, on physical and mental health. Ayurvedic practitioners believe in the healing power of nature, the importance of treating the whole person, and the prevention of illness as the ultimate cure.

Sushruta, an Ayurvedic healer who lived four thousand years ago, defined a healthy person as, "He [who is] in balance, whose digestion, assimilation, and metabolism are good, whose tissues and wastes are created properly, and whose self, mind, and senses remain full of bliss" (Fein, 124).

Ayurvedic practitioners evaluate all aspects of a patient's life to determine the person's mind/body type, or *dosha*. Health is achieved when the dosha is brought into balance through diet, lifestyle, and exercise. The senses can also affect the dosha. Therefore, Ayurvedic doctors might suggest relaxing music, aromatherapy, massage, or spending time outdoors.

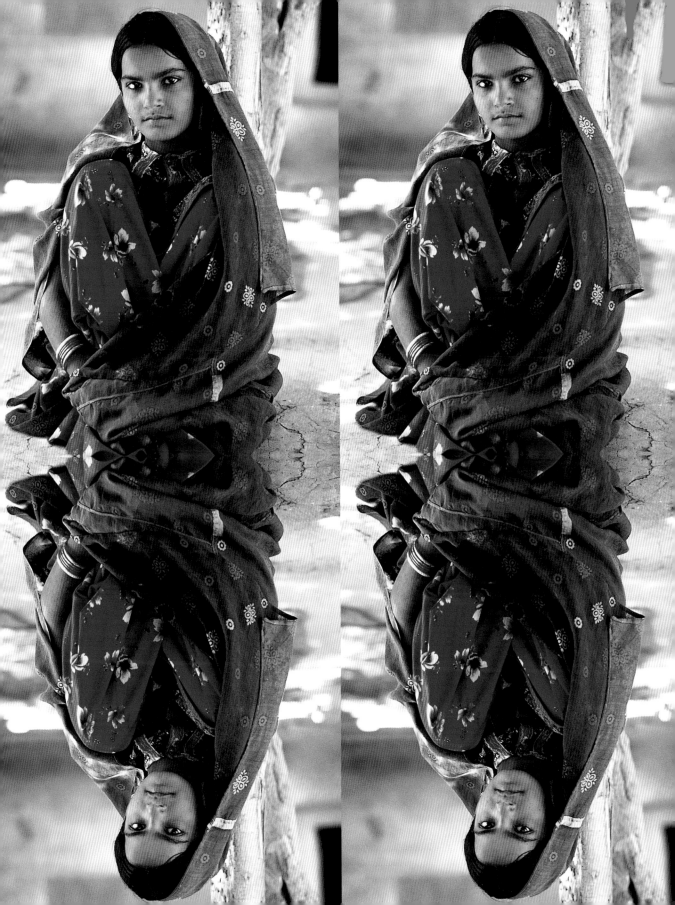

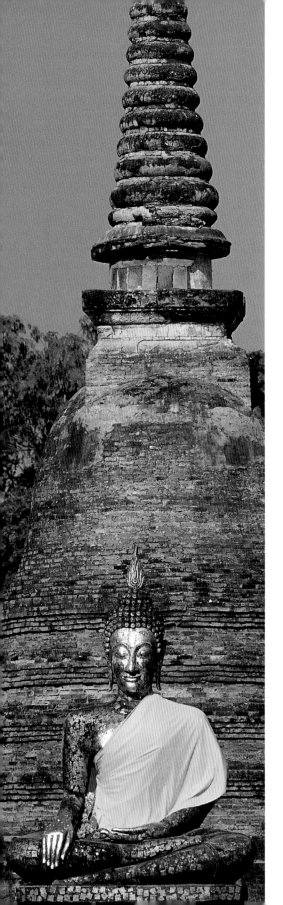

The Healing Power of Faith

Acts of ritual and prayer are primary components of the healing process in virtually all cultures. For example, the ancient Egyptians prayed to Imhotep, the sacred healer; the Greeks had Asclepius; and Christians found healing through Jesus Christ and various saints. Whether a person believes in a specific divinity or simply believes that there is a higher force or universal energy, the healing power of faith cannot be denied.

Whatever one's religious affiliation (or lack thereof), since prayer is a way of meditating, its effects are similar to those of other kinds of meditation: focusing and quieting the mind, slowing the heart rate, reducing blood pressure, and lowering levels of stress-related hormones that can weaken immune function.

For the first time since religion and science parted ways in Western culture in the seventeenth century, the healing power of prayer is being recognized by the medical community. Medical research is demonstrating that spirituality is an important tool that can greatly improve a patient's course of recovery (Faneuil, 46).

FAITH IS THE OPENING OF ALL SIDES AND
EVERY LEVEL OF ONE'S LIFE TO THE DIVINE INFLOW.

MARTIN LUTHER KING, JR.
American, 20th century

Life Force

The underlying premise of many ancient holistic healing practices is that health and well-being come from proper nurturing and direction of the vital energy or life force that is at the core of all living things. In Chinese tradition this energy is known as *chi*, in Japan it is *ki*, in India it is *prana*.

When life force flows smoothly and freely, body and mind are in health and harmony, and the body's organs can function properly. If the energy is blocked, illness can occur. Therefore, various Eastern medical techniques (see boxes below) call for unblocking the body's energy. These methods can relieve ailments ranging from headaches to heart disease, depression to diabetes (Colino, 49).

In Eastern medical tradition, many healing arts are forms of therapeutic touch involving the stimulation of certain key points on the body.

A trained practitioner can manipulate the body's energy so that the chi can be redirected, relieving anxiety, pain, and disease.

Methods for bringing the dosha into balance:
- *Get more sleep: go to bed early and wake up early.*
- *Eat the main meal of the day at noon and a lighter meal at night.*
- *Choose fresh, whole foods (organic if possible), eat simply, and follow a vegetarian diet, or a modified vegetarian diet that includes some fish and/or chicken.*
- *Cleanse the system monthly by eating only vegetables and whole grains for a day or two.*
- *Meditate daily.*
- *Spend time outdoors as often as possible.*

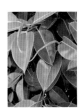

ACUPUNCTURE

THIS TREATMENT STIMULATES THE BODY'S ENERGY USING EXTREMELY THIN NEEDLES INSERTED INTO SPECIFIC POINTS ON THE BODY.

MOXIBUSTION

USING HEAT FROM SLOW-BURNING STICKS MADE OF HERBS ON ACUPUNCTURE POINTS, MOXIBUSTION ENHANCES THE EFFECTS OF ACUPUNCTURE.

ACUPRESSURE

THERAPISTS APPLY PRESSURE TO SPECIFIC POINTS ON THE BODY TO INCREASE BLOOD CIRCULATION AND TO RELEASE ENDORPHINS, THE BODY'S NATURAL PAINKILLERS.

SHIATSU

THIS TECHNIQUE INVOLVES MORE RIGOROUS MASSAGING OF THE PRESSURE POINTS.

REIKI

THE LAYING ON OF HANDS IS INTENDED TO MANIPULATE THE PATIENT'S BODY ENERGY.

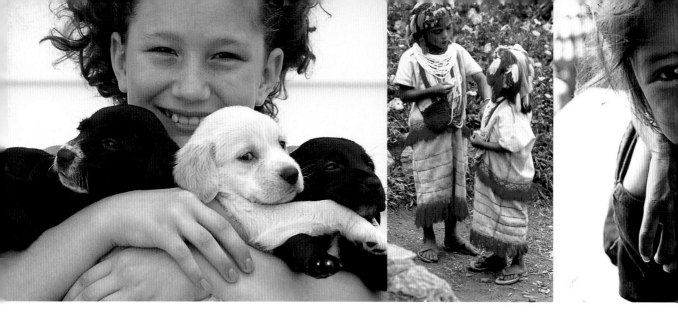

ALL YOU NEED IS LOVE.
LOVE IS ALL YOU NEED.

JOHN LENNON
English, 20th century
from *"All You Need Is Love"*

THE HEALING POWER OF LOVE

The miracles of the modern world have caused people to be literally and figuratively out of touch with each other. People live more solitary lives, communicating via wires, cables, or cyberspace, rather than face to face. Despite labor-saving devices, Americans work more hours than ever before. That leaves less time for friends, family, and social functions.

By contrast, many indigenous cultures rely on tribal connections for their very survival. A person's extended family provides food, shelter, care for children and the elderly, and protection from outside enemies.

Loneliness is a powerful toxin. Social isolation is a major source of stress, and stress produces an unhealthy domino effect: hyperarousal of the autonomic nervous system over time impairs the immune system, making you more vulnerable to infections and other diseases (Ornish, 43).

The immune system receives some of its most significant neural input from the emotional center of the brain. Thus, isolation and suppressed emotions can often lead to illness, while intimacy and social support can heal.

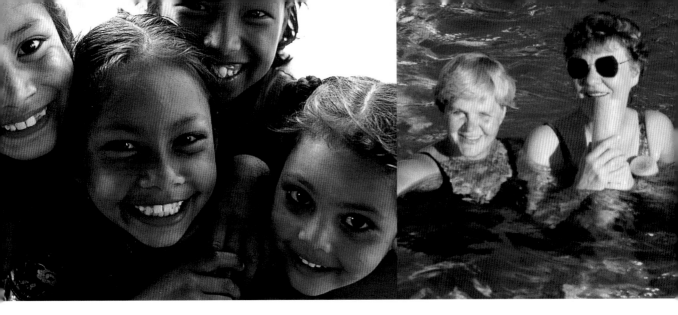

TELL ME WHO ADMIRES AND LOVES YOU,
AND I WILL TELL YOU WHO YOU ARE.

CHARLES AUGUSTINE SAINTE-BEUVE
French, 19th century

Some things to consider:

- A major study reported that social isolation is as significant a factor in mortality rates as smoking, high blood pressure, high cholesterol, obesity, and lack of physical exercise.

- People with few or weak social relationships have been shown to be at twice the risk of dying from heart attacks as those with strong social ties.

- A Stanford University study of women with advanced breast cancer demonstrated that women who participated in weekly support groups in addition to conventional therapy had a better chance of survival after five years than those who had therapy alone.

- Research shows that people who have a network of friends, strong family ties, or a relationship with a significant other have a lower risk of dying from heart disease, cancer, and other conditions than people who are socially isolated.

- A Yale University study of heart patients found that patients who felt the most love and support had less severe obstruction of the arteries than those who felt less loved.   *(from Rhodes)*

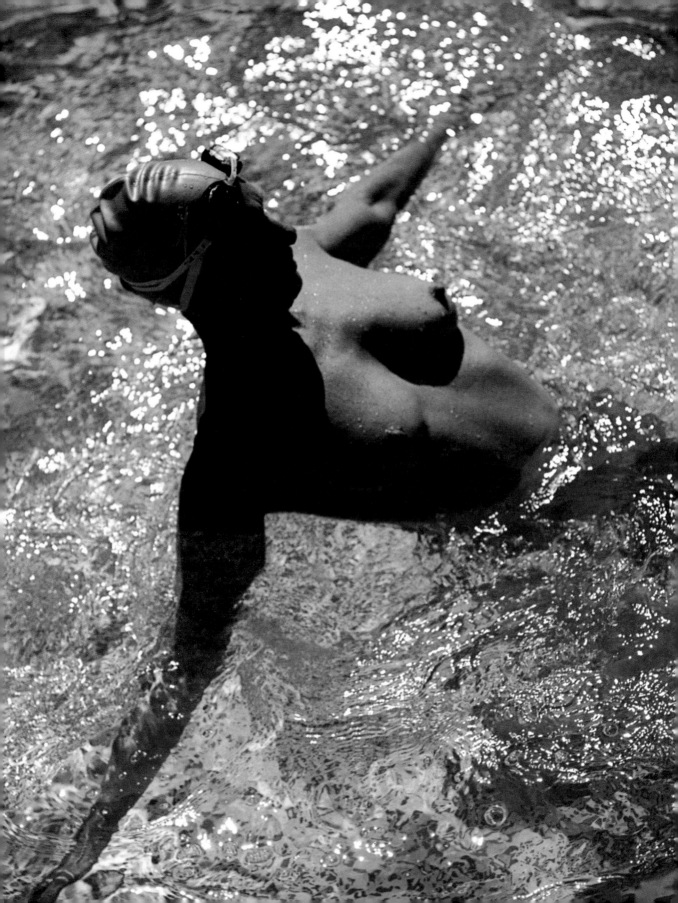

Fitness

The physically active woman that we associate with modern times is really nothing new. Artemis was the Greek goddess of hunting and fertility. Her counterpart in Roman mythology was Diana, huntress and perennial virgin. Both were fit, vital, "outdoorsy" deities, known for their wisdom and independence. In Edmund Spenser's sixteenth-century chivalric epic *The Faerie Queene,* Britomart (whose name is derived from an attendant of Artemis) is a female knight who wields her sword mightily against beast and foe.

No shrinking violets here: they are strong, vigorous, and beautiful feminine personae. Today, just as then, an active, healthy body is a beautiful body. Exercise can strengthen the heart, muscles, and bones, improving endurance, flexibility, and coordination. Exercise has also been shown to lead to clearer thinking and better moods. The boost it gives to blood circulation benefits skin, hair, and nails, providing important nutrients and processing wastes and toxins more efficiently.

Although many women in developed countries are active in their daily lives, the rigors of family, job, and home, exhausting though they might be, do not include the most beneficial kinds of exercise. In general terms, most women can benefit from a program that includes two types of exercise: aerobic and weight-bearing.

Aerobic exercise. This type of exercise is characterized by increased respiration and heart rate. In developing countries, women plow fields, wash clothes and utensils by hand, hike to mountain meadows with their herds, beat grain into flour—all high-energy activities.

For those of us who live relatively sedentary lives, aerobic exercise can include running, brisk walking, dancing, tennis, cross-country skiing, swimming, and stair climbing. These are all excellent ways to improve cardiopulmonary function and increase endurance.

Weight-bearing exercise. This type of exercise puts pressure on muscles and bones. It has been demonstrated that weight-bearing exercise causes bones to become thicker and stronger. This is especially important in warding off osteoporosis.

If you are not used to carrying large urns of water on your head or loads of firewood on your back, weightlifting or exercising with weights (like walking with hand weights) will help build bone and muscle strength.

In addition, a balanced fitness regimen includes stretching. Stretching should always accompany any vigorous workout: beforehand, to loosen up, and afterward, to cool down. Stretching can also be done in the morning to help you wake up, in the evening to help the body relax, or anytime during the day to relieve tension and reinvigorate yourself. Yoga (see page 157) is an intense stretching regimen that can also be worked in to your daily routine.

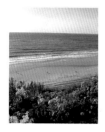
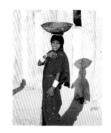

IT TAKES ALL THE RUNNING YOU CAN DO, TO KEEP IN THE SAME PLACE.
IF YOU WANT TO GET SOMEWHERE ELSE,
YOU MUST RUN AT LEAST TWICE AS FAST AS THAT!

LEWIS CARROLL
English, 19th century
from *Through the Looking-Glass*

Get with the Program

Alice is not the only female to be run off her feet. The good news is that to maintain fitness, prolonged, strenuous exercise is not necessary. Moderate exercise every day, such as 30 minutes of brisk walking, is a great way to keep in shape. Any activity is better than none. Walking is better than sitting.

The only good exercise plan is one that is enjoyable. The best way to get enough exercise is to integrate it into a regular schedule. If exercise is part of a daily routine, it becomes a pleasure rather than a chore. A regular schedule does not mean you must do exactly the same kind of exercise at exactly the same time of day (unless you prefer that). Try varying the routine to keep things interesting. Be flexible; don't berate yourself for missing a day now and then.

Look for other ways to add physical activity to your day. Take the stairs instead of the elevator. Bike to work. Don't have phone meetings; instead, walk down the hall and talk to colleagues in person. Park farther away from your destination, and walk an extra quar-ter mile each way. Go out dancing.

Too often these days exercise means riding a stationary bike while reading a newspaper in a room full of sweaty people. Exercise is not only a way to get in tune with the body, it's also an opportunity to connect with nature. Walk on the beach. Head for the hills on a mountain bike. Cross-country ski in the park. Run in the woods. Climb every mountain. Take a dip in the lake (better for skin, hair, and eyes than a chlorinated pool).

Even urban denizens can take advantage of the great outdoors. Air quality indoors is often much worse than even a congested city street at rush hour. This is especially true of health clubs whose windows are often sealed shut, and whose ventilation systems recycle air that contains bacteria, mold, mildew, and fumes from cleaning products, chlorine, plastics, glues, and paints—not to mention air used by vast numbers of perspiring people.

Exercise is a chance to escape, to quit the confines of four walls and everyday routine. Exercising outdoors increases the sensation of getting away. It's a chance to clear the mind of

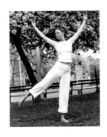 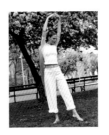

HEAVEN, I'M IN HEAVEN, AND MY HEART BEATS SO THAT I CAN HARDLY SPEAK,
AND I SEEM TO FIND THE HAPPINESS I SEEK
WHEN WE'RE OUT TOGETHER DANCING CHEEK TO CHEEK.

IRVING BERLIN
American, born Russian, 20th century
from "Cheek to Cheek"

daily clutter, making room for thoughtful consideration of the changing color of the leaves, or an unusual bird song, or the scent of the grass after a rainstorm.

Music and Dance

Whether you find paradise waltzing to Strauss or moshing to Nirvana, when dancing, you are engaging in an interplay of motion and emotion that has accompanied ecstatic and healing rituals in many parts of the world since before recorded history. Cave paintings depict human figures in solemn or celebratory motion. In some parts of Africa, the *malam* (spiritual healer) uses therapeutic touch combined with music and dance to ward off the evil spirits that plague the sick.

Dance is a physical experience that stimulates the senses and encourages emotional expression. It inspires creativity, fosters a sense of the whole self, and promotes feelings of well-being. Many cultures incorporate natural imagery into dance movements, evoking the motion of a river, the wind, an animal.

Evidence suggests that dance and song preceded speech—music may truly be our native tongue. Beyond its value as art or entertainment, music has a powerful effect on our brain, and thus on our health. It is a connection made in many cultures. In Greek mythology, Apollo was the god of both music and healing. In Japan, doctors have been known to prescribe a dose of Mendelssohn's "Spring Song" or Dvorak's "Humoresque" for migraine sufferers.

Although many types of music can be calming, the work of Mozart is particularly effective. Studies have found that, regardless of the subjects' personal tastes or cultural backgrounds, listening to Mozart is soothing, improves listeners' spatial perceptions, and allows them to express themselves more clearly. Listening to Mozart before an IQ test can boost scores by roughly nine points (Westley and Gideonse, 103). This phenomenon, dubbed the Mozart effect, is not limited to human subjects. In monasteries in Brittany, French monks have observed that cows that listen to Mozart give more milk.

Nutrition

Twenty-four hundred years ago, Hippocrates suggested that self-knowledge was the best approach to better living, and today, prevention is still the best prescription for beauty and well-being. Eating a balanced diet of natural foods and drinking liberal amounts of water are simple ways to keep healthy and beautiful.

In earlier eras, people ate whatever they could; starvation was (and for half the world, still is) a much more pressing problem than obesity. In many ways, our bodies are still hard-wired for times of privation. The craving for salt, for instance, is the vestige of an era when hunter-gatherers had difficulty finding enough salt, vital to proper metabolism, for their diet.

The perfect body is a myth that's not worth chasing. What you might choose to pursue instead are sane, healthy habits based on sound principles of nutrition.

You Are What You Eat

It doesn't take a Gallic genius to understand that whatever works its way through the gastrointestinal system will eventually have an effect on the rest of the body. It makes sense that the more closely foods resemble the body's chemical makeup, the more easily the body can process and use them.

Unfortunately, many foods on shelves or fast-food counters are full of useless, and in some cases harmful, ingredients—many of which are not included on the label. Fruits and vegetables that have been sprayed with chemical pesticides do not have those "ingredients" listed; milk from cows treated with bovine growth hormone (rBGH) is not required to be so labeled; companies that feed their chickens antibiotics don't usually advertise it on their packaging.

The idea is not to become hyper-vigilant about every molecule you put into your body, but rather to understand that many foods contain substances that you do not need, the safety of which is uncertain.

Why worry, if these products and practices are approved by the FDA? For one thing, the FDA is not infallible. In a recent example, pressure from medical and consumer watchdog groups prompted the FDA to reconsider its guidelines for antibiotics (used as growth enhancers) in animal feed. Studies done by the Centers for Disease Control and Prevention have shown a disturbing link between the overuse of antibiotics in animal feed and an increase in strains of antibiotic-resistant bacteria. Using these antibiotics to grow a bigger chicken may render an entire class of drugs useless in fighting the diseases they were originally designed to treat.

Even substances that appear safe in studies may not be harmless to every individual. Certain segments of the population are routinely excluded from medical testing. For example, producers and users of rBGH say studies find no adverse effects from its consumption; however, those studies rarely, if ever, include children, who are, of course, major milk drinkers. Consider how a glass of wine, which wouldn't make the

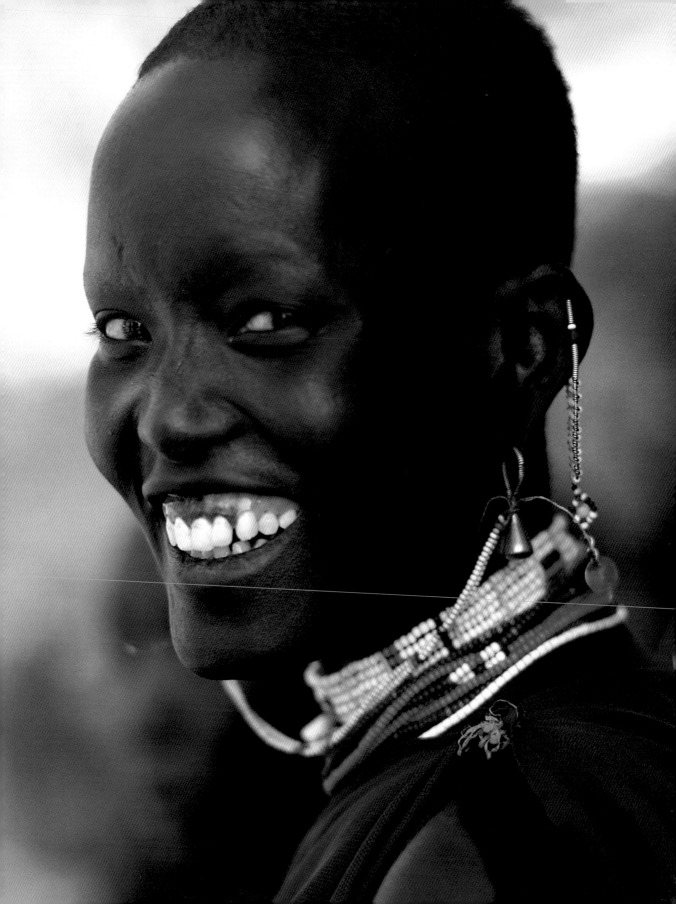

average adult feel tipsy, could make a toddler very sick.

A concentration of chemicals acceptable in adults may cause serious problems in children, in the elderly, in people of a particular ethnic group, or in pregnant and nursing women. Safety studies often do not trace the cumulative effect of chemical additives over time, or in combination with other chemicals, or in relation to chronic conditions like hypertension or diabetes.

The moral is, take food safety claims with a grain of salt.

DO I DARE TO EAT A PEACH?
T. S. ELIOT
American, 20th century
from "The Love Song of J. Alfred Prufrock"

Don't Panic, Try Organic

A simple solution to this problem is to choose foods that have no chemical additives from growing, processing, or packaging. Buy organic. Organic farming is based on the principle that healthy soil is naturally rich, and healthy plants are naturally resistant to pests and disease. After all, farmers have been using all-natural techniques for tens of thousands of years, and they have developed effective fertilizing and pest control methods that don't rely on synthetic agents.

Organic products may cost more than conventionally grown products, as they cost more to produce. However, since organic foods are not treated with preservatives, they tend to be sold locally; so by buying organic, you are often supporting small-scale farmers who are dedicated to preserving the regional environment. If we believe in the interconnectedness of all things, of man with all of

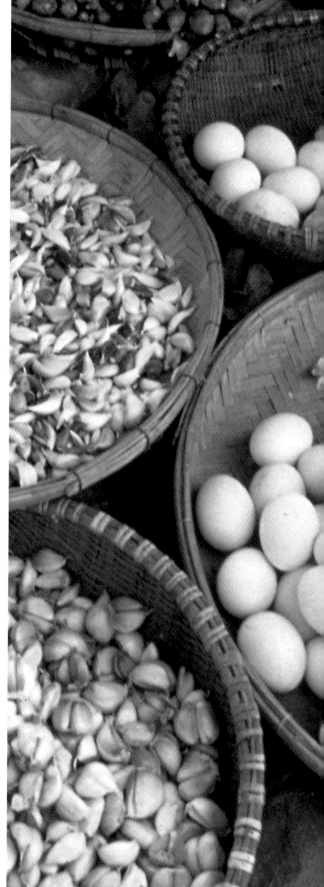

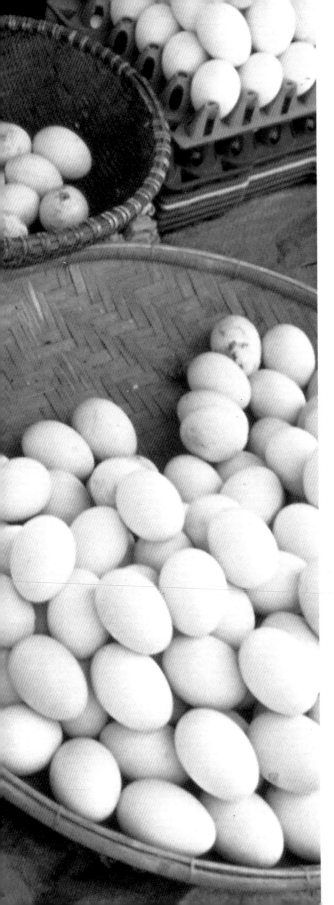

nature, something that's bad for the earth cannot be good for the body. Equally as important, organic produce tastes better.

The Genuine, Certified Miracle Diet

Eat a variety of foods, with an emphasis on grains, fruits, and vegetables. The diets of most indigenous cultures tend to be high in carbohydrates, low in sugars and fats. The exception is found among arctic and subarctic peoples. Their rich-in-fat diets are a vital adaptation to cold climates, where extra calories are needed.

For anyone not chasing down caribou in subzero temperatures, yellow and green leafy vegetables are essential. They are full of a variety of vitamins and minerals beneficial to skin, hair, and nails. Grains supply carbohydrates—most of the sugars your body needs—and roughage. Fresh fruit is a major source of vitamins and fiber.

It is only relatively recently in humankind's evolutionary history that man has been eating game, and our gastrointestinal system's ability to process meat has not quite caught up to our ability to procure large quantities of it. Meat can also be loaded with chemicals and with toxic bacteria from improper processing, handling, and preparation. Seek out organic, free-range meat products whenever possible. Eat meat in moderation.

There is speculation that trace elements in whole foods aid the body in utilizing vitamins and minerals more efficiently. In addition, the vital substances in foodstuffs are more readily available to, and more easily absorbed by, the body than those found in synthetic supplements. You can't eat junk food all day, pop a vitamin pill, and expect that it will right all nutritional wrongs. Supplements should supplement, not be substituted for, a rich and varied diet.

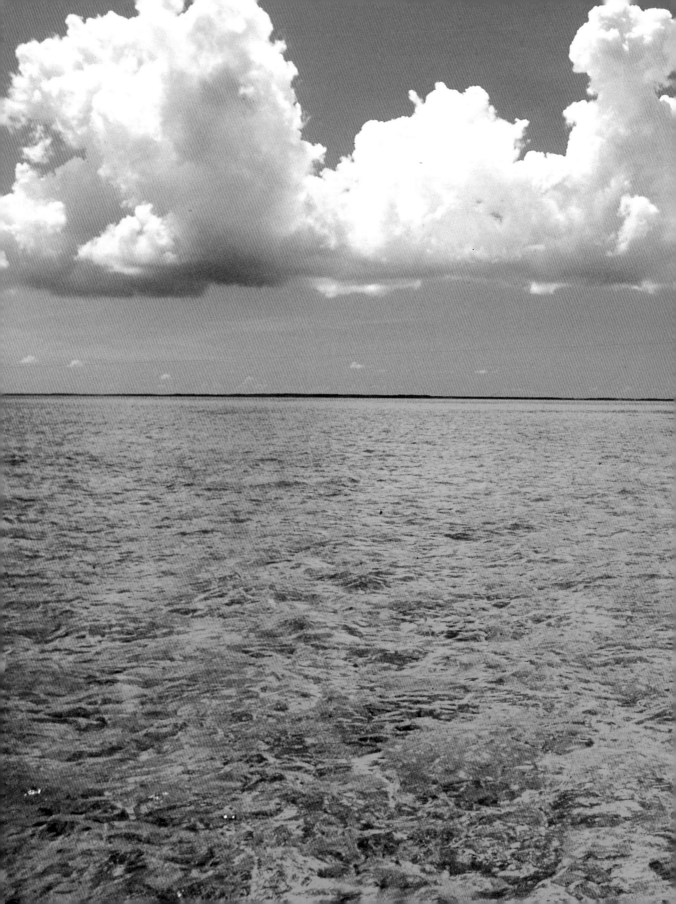

WATER: THE ESSENCE OF LIFE

Water is the most important ingredient in health and beauty. Hardly surprising, considering that the human body is approximately 70 percent water—accounting for about half of a woman's weight. The average person needs between eight and ten eight-ounce glasses of water daily, and even more during illness, strenuous exercise, or really hot weather.

Water runs the body's vital systems, literally, keeping everything in balance. Water is responsible for establishing homeostasis, which means that water preserves a uniform, stable state between interdependent biochemical and physiological processes. Water also maintains a balance in osmotic pressure, which is the physical force that keeps certain elements on one side of the cell membrane from moving across the membrane. Without water, your cells would collapse. Water-borne electrolytes insure that minimal changes occur in the acid-base balance of the body's fluids. If they became too alkaline or acidic, the basic processes that keep you alive would simply shut down.

Water is essential to beautiful skin, hair, nails, and body. It is vital for circulation, bringing nutrients to, and transporting wastes from, epidermal cells. Drinking lots of water can fight dry skin, dull, lifeless hair, and brittle, cracked nails.

It's a myth that water retention is a cause or symptom of obesity. On the contrary, overweight people have a lower ratio of body water to body weight than people of average weight. Athletes, especially endurance athletes, tend to have the highest percentage of water to body weight.

There is no substitute for water. Juices are higher in sugar content and lower in fiber than the fruits they come from. Sodas are loaded with chemicals, which actually increase thirst. Alcohol and caffeine are diuretics that can raise water-intake requirements. Aside from drinking water, a diet full of fruits and vegetables (which contain 70 to 90 percent water) is a delicious way to boost your intake.

Of course the best way to insure a good water supply for all is not to pollute and to avoid products that do. Water was sacred to virtually every preindustrial culture. Gods and spirits were believed to inhabit water sources, and to defile them was considered a grave sin.

It still is. Use water sparingly. Avoid harsh soaps and detergents. Buy organic foods produced without chemical pesticides and fertilizers that contaminate ground water. Recycle whenever possible, so waste products won't go into landfill and leach into the water supply.

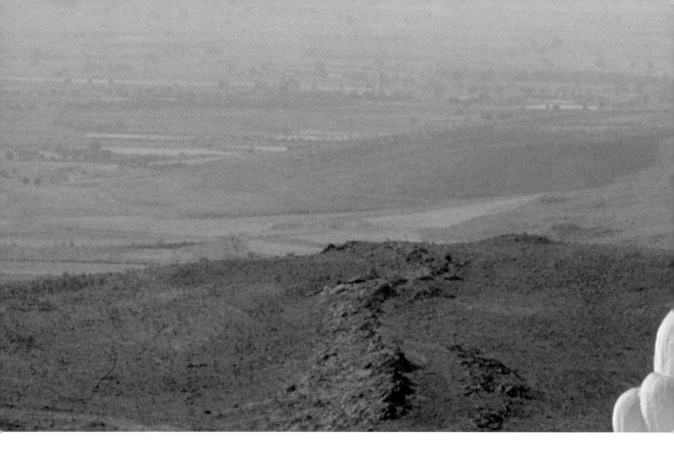

The Balance of Nature

Much of Western literature and art emphasizes the conflict between man and nature. Eastern and indigenous cultures, in contrast, see man as a part of, not standing in opposition to, nature. As creatures of the natural world, appreciating our connection to nature and experiencing its sensory delights can bring a sense of calm, peace, serenity, and well-being.

People are profoundly influenced by communion with the natural world. Gazing upon a wide-open vista, for example, can be relaxing during the winter months because it counteracts the tension caused by being in enclosed spaces. Time at the beach lends itself to meditation and deep breathing, which can reflect the rhythmic sounds of the surf and the repetitive motion of the waves.

There are many ways to reconnect with nature, even if most of your waking hours are spent in a cubicle. When you can't go strolling on the beach or hiking in the mountains, you can still reap some benefits by surrounding yourself with pictures of nature. Post photographs of favorite landscapes around your work area. When stress and tension set in, take a moment

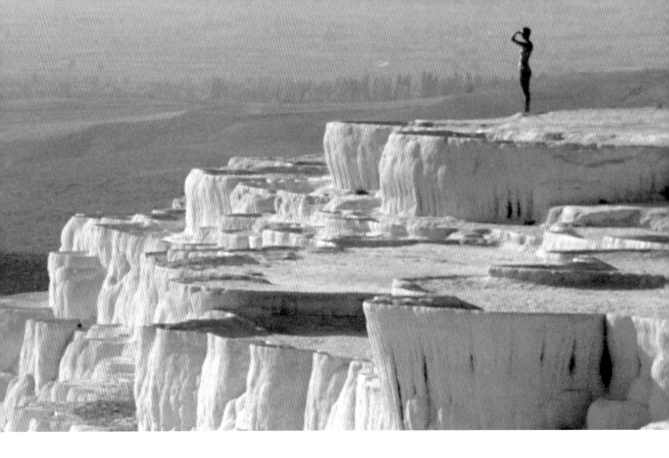

OH WORLD, I CANNOT HOLD THEE CLOSE ENOUGH.

EDNA ST. VINCENT MILLAY
American, 20th century

to breathe deeply, and visualize yourself walking through that landscape. Imagine what you would see, hear, smell, and feel.

When you can get outside, find a quiet, private place, and close your eyes; breathing deeply, carefully attend to the sensations around you. As you begin to walk, keep your eyes closed and take notice of the heightened sense of sound, smell, and touch that is possible when vision is absent. As you walk, meditate on your breathing and visualize the process by which plants release the oxygen you inhale, and breathe in the carbon dioxide

you exhale. Sense the perfect balance of this symbiosis. Imagine your breath as it flows out into nature, giving life to herbs, grass, and trees.

As you open your eyes, take time to focus on a particular object—a flower, a tree branch, a mossy stone—and notice the details you never would have seen if you had walked by quickly. Combine this observation with meditational breathing.

As you become more aware of the balance of the natural world, it will be easier to understand and appreciate the natural balance of mind, body, and spirit in all human beings.

RESOURCES

If you have questions or comments, or you'd like to share a recipe, please feel free to contact me at my website, www.dawngallagher.com.
The companies listed below carry all-natural beauty products.

NATUROPATHICA
74 Montauk Highway
East Hampton, NY 11937
1-800-669-7618

BORNEO BASICS
www.dawngallagher.com
1-800-373-7475

THE NATURAL DENTIST/WOODSTOCK
NATURAL PRODUCTS
Englewood Cliffs, NJ 07632
1-800-615-6895

WELEDA, INC.
P.O. Box 249
Congers, NY 10092
800-289-1969

AUBREY ORGANICS
Tampa, FL 33614
800-AUBREY-H

PHILLIP KINGSLEY HAIR CARE TRI-
CHOLOGICAL CENTRE
16 East 53rd Street
New York, NY 10022

ZIA
San Francisco, 94107
800-334-7516

DR. E. H. BONNER AND ASSOC.
Box 28
Escondido, CA 92030
706-743-2211

COMMON SENSE
109 Lincoln Avenue
Rutland, VT 802-773-0582

WILD HILL HERBALS
RR1 Box 212A
Chelsea, VT 06503

SUNSHINE
Eugene, OR 97402
800-225-3623

LAKON HERBALS
Box 252
Montpelier, VT 05601
800-TO-LAKON

BURT'S BEES
Raleigh, NC 27612
800-849-7112

LILY OF THE DESERT
Irving, TX 75063

TISSERAND
Avalon Natural Cosmetics
Petaluma, CA 94975-0428

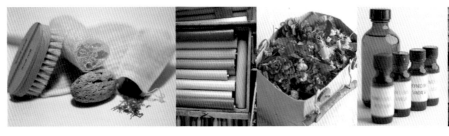
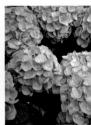

VERMONT SOAPWORKS
76 Exchange Street
Middlebury, VT 05753
802-388-4302

CLOUDWORKS
Contoocook, NH 03229

PURPLE CONEFLOWER
Riverside Farm
RR1 Box 80
East Hardwick, VT 05836

GREEN MOUNTAIN HERBS
P.O. Box 532
Putney, VT 05346

AURA CACIA
Weaverville, CA 96093
www.auracacia.com

RIVER SOAP COMPANY
1078 Illinois Street
San Francisco, CA 94107

ORGANIC SKIN CARE
OOVO COSMETICS
PO Box 606
Hoboken, NJ 07030
1-800-996-6686

BEAUTY WITHOUT CRUELTY
Petaluma, CA 94975-0428

DR. HAUSHKA
59C North Street
Hatfield, MA 01038
1-800-247-9907

ESSENTIAL OILS
Frontier Aromatherapy
www.frontiercoop.com
1-800-786-1388

NATURE'S ALCHEMY/LOTUS BRANDS
POB 325
Twin Lakes, WI 53181

BACH FLOWERS
Flower Essence Energy/Maggie Smith
3732 Crete Street
San Diego, CA
619-581-3839

NATRACARE
Denver, CO 80206

ORGANIC ESSENTIALS
RT. 1 Box 120
O'Donnell, TX 79351

CONSERVATION INTERNATIONAL
2501 M Street N.W., Suite 200
Washington, DC 20037
1-800-406-2306
www.conservation.org

BIBLIOGRAPHY

Aero, Rita. *The Complete Book of Longevity.* New York: Perigee Books, 1980.

Batterberry, Michael, and Ariane Batterberry. *Fashion: The Mirror of History.* New York: Greenwich House, 1982.

Benet, William Rose. *The Reader's Encyclopedia.* New York: Thomas Y. Crowell, Publishers, 1965.

Bletcher, Michele Brown. "Play Hard, Breathe Deeply: Can an Ancient Method of Breath Control Help You Function Better, Faster, and Longer—and Stay Healthier Too?," *Women's Sports and Fitness* 19, no. 2 (March 1997), 52.

Boorstin, Daniel J. *The Discoverers.* New York: Vintage, 1985.

Boston Women's Health Collective. *The New Our Bodies, Ourselves.* New York: Touchstone Books, 1992.

Braudel, Fernand. *The Structures of Everyday Life.* New York: Harper & Row, 1981.

———. *The Wheels of Commerce.* New York: Harper & Row, 1982.

———. *The Perspective of the World.* New York: Harper & Row, 1984.

Brody, Jane. *Jane Brody's* The New York Times *Guide to Personal Health.* New York: Times Books, 1982.

Buchman, Dian Dincin. *Herbal Medicine.* New York: Gramercy Publishing Company, 1979.

Burenhult, Goran, ed. *Traditional Peoples Today.* New York: Harper Collins, 1994.

Burger, Julian. *The Gaia Atlas of First Peoples.* London: Gaia Books, Ltd., 1990.

Busch, Julia. *The Home Guide to Natural Beauty Care.* New York: Berkley Books, 1995.

Campbell, Joseph. *The Power of Myth.* New York: Doubleday, 1988.

Cox, Janice. *Natural Beauty at Home: More Than 200 Easy-to-Use Recipes for Body, Bath, and Hair.* New York: Henry Holt and Company, 1994.

Colino, Stacey. "Harness the Energy," *Women's Sports and Fitness* 18, no. 8 (Nov.-Dec. 1996): 44(5).

Curtis, Susan, Romy Fraser, and Irene Kohler. *Neal's Yard Natural Remedies.* London: Arkana/Penguin, 1988.

De Bonneville, Françoise. *The Book of the Bath.* New York: Rizzoli, 1998.

Dennee, JoAnne. *In the Three Sisters Garden.* Montpelier, VT: Food Works/Common Roots Press, 1995.

Denslow, Julie Sloan, and Christine Padoch, eds. *People of the Tropical Rainforest.* Berkeley: University of California Press, 1988.

Densmore, Frances. *How Indians Used Wild Plants for Food, Medicine and Crafts.* New York: Dover, 1974.

Diamond, Harvey, and Marilyn Diamond. *Fit for Life.* New York: Warner Books, 1987.

Elkington, John, Julia Hailes, and Joel Makower. *The Green Consumer.* New York: Penguin Books, 1990.

Faneuil, Nichole. "The Spirituality of Wellness: Physicians Say Religious Belief Contributes to Healing," *American Fitness* 15, no. 6 (Nov.-Dec. 1997): 42 (5).

Fein, Jessica. "Which Natural Medicine is for You?," *Natural Health* 27, no. 2 (March-April 1998) 119 (10).

Fischer-Rizzi, Susanne. *Complete Aromatherapy Handbook.* New York: Sterling Publishing Company, 1990.

Gilmore, Melvin. *Uses of Plants by the Indians of the Upper Missouri River Region.* Lincoln: University of Nebraska Press, 1991.

Gladstar, Rosemary. *Herbal Healing for Women*. New York: Fireside Books, 1993.

Guyton, Anita. *The Natural Beauty Book*. London: HarperCollins, 1991.

Hale, Judson, ed. *The Best of The Old Farmer's Almanac*. New York: Random House, 1991.

Hampton, Aubrey. *Natural Organic Hair and Skin Care*. Florida: Organica Press, 1987.

Harp, David, and Nina Feldman. "3 Minutes to Total Relaxation," *Prevention* 49, no. 9 (Sept. 1997) 148 (6).

Harris, Jessica. *The World Beauty Book*. New York: HarperCollins, 1995.

Harvard Medical School. *Vitamins and Minerals*. Cambridge: Harvard Medical School Health Publications Group, 1995.

Heinerman, John. *The Encyclopededia of Healing Juices*. New York: Parker Publishing Company, 1994.

Holmes, George, ed. *The Oxford Illustrated History of Medieval Europe*. New York: Oxford University Press, 1992.

Huizinga, Johan. *The Autumn of the Middle Ages*. Chicago: University of Chicago Press, 1996.

Kent, Debra. "Meditation Hits the Mainstream," *Cosmopolitan* 219, no. 2 (August 1995): 194 (4).

Kingsley, Phillip. *Hair: An Owners Handbook*. London: Aurum Press Limited, 1995.

Langman, Jan, M.D. and Martin W. Woerdeman, M.D. *Atlas of Medical Anatomy*. Philadelphia: The Saunders Press, 1982.

Lawless, Julia. *The Illustrated Encyclopedia of Essential Oils*. Rockport, Mass.: Element Books, Inc., 1995.

Ornish, Dean, MD. *Love & Survival: The Scientific Basis for the Healing Power of Intimacy*. New York: HarperCollins, 1998.

Melpomene Institute for Women's Health Research. *The Bodywise Woman*. Champaign, Ill.: Human Kinetics Publishers, 1990.

Milne, Lorus J., and Margery Milne. *Living Plants of the World*. New York: Random House, 1987.

Northrup, Christiane, MD. *Women's Bodies, Women's Wisdom*. New York: Bantam Books, 1998.

Rector Page, Linda, MD., PhD. *Healthy Healing: A Guide to Self-Healing for Everyone*. California: Healthy Healing Publications, 1997.

Rhodes, Elizabeth. "Rx for Good Health: Intimacy," *Seattletimes.com* (March 25, 1998).

Runkel, Sylvan T., and Dean M. Roosa. *Wildflowers of the Tallgrass Prairie: The Upper Midwest*. Ames: Iowa State University Press, 1988.

Shangold, Mona, and Gabe Mirkin. *The Complete Sports Medicine Book for Women*. New York: Fireside Books, 1985.

Shosteck, Robert. *Flowers and Plants*. New York: Quadrangle/The New York Times Book Company, 1974.

Silver, Helene. *The Body-Smart System*. New York: Bantam Books, 1990.

Sinnige, Jacqueline. *Spiritual Beauty Care*. Twin Lakes, Wis.: Lotus Press, 1997.

Weiss, Gaea, and Shandor Weiss. *Growing & Using the Healing Herbs*. New York: Wing Books, 1992.

Westley, Marian, and Ted Gideonse. "Music is Good Medicine," *Newsweek* 132, no. 12 (Sept. 21, 1998): 103 (1).

"Yoga: The Ultimate Mind-Body Workout," *Harvard Health Letter* 24, no. 2 (Dec. 1, 1998): n/a.

CONTRIBUTORS

Photography ~ Bill Cardoni

Still life and how-to photography ~ David Webber

Contributing photography ~

Dimitri Halkidis, Waring Abbott, Bud Struck, Pauline St. Denis, Meghan Boody

Design and art direction~ Ronni Ascagni

Design assistant- Patricia Stein

Photo editing ~ Jenny Bunker Cardoni, Ronni Ascagni

Makeup and hair ~ Jo-Ann DiLorenzo

Stylist ~ Barbra Jerard

Models~

Francine Tint, Claudine Thomas, Mila Radulavic, Baret Boisson

Research ~

Tara Milutis and Susan Blinkhorn

Bill Cardoni: page 18 all, 26, 30, 31, 33, 41, 46, 50, 52, 55 center and bottom, 56 center (banana), 57, 58 left and right, 61 right, 62, 65, 68 top and bottom, 69, 76 left, 78, 79, 81, 84 center, 88, 89, 93, 97, 100, 101, 104 right, 105 right, 115 left and right, 117, 119, 120 bottom, 123, 129, 136 left, 148 left, 156 top, 157, 161, 167, 168, 169, 170, 171 left, 173, 174 all, 177, 178–9, 180, 182–3

Dimitri Halkidis: page 6, 8, 21, 23, 24–5, 35, 42, 59, 60 right, 80, 95 center, 99, 112, 124 left, 128, 130 center and bottom, 132–3, 134, 155, 158 all, 162 left, 163, 175

David Webber: page 2, 20, 22, 27, 28, 29, 32, 34 bottom, 36 left, 39, 45, 49, 56 all except center, 58 center, 60 left, 61 left, 68 center, 71 bottom, 74, 75, 76 right, 77 all, 82, 84 left and right, 86, 87 all, 90, 96, 98, 102, 105 left, 106 all, 109, 110 all, 118, 120 right and left, 121, 122, 124 right, 137 all, 140, 141 all, 142 all, 143, 145 all, 146, 147, 148 right, 149 center and right, 150 all, 152 all, 156 bottom, 162 center and right, 185 all except right

Dawn Gallagher: page 34 top, 36 right, 37 right, 43, 55 top, 71 top, 83, 95 top and bottom, 104 left, 111, 120 center, 124 center, 149 left, 156 center, 185 right

Pauline St. Denis: page 37 left

Bud Struck: page 17, 73, 115 center, 127

Waring Abbott: page 67, 172

Meghan Boody: page 164

ACKNOWLEDGMENTS

My love and appreciation go to all my family and friends
around the world who contributed information and recipes for this book.
To my beautiful mother, Dorothy Gallagher, and my sisters, Doreen and Deborah.

I would also like to sincerely thank everyone who contributed
their time and efforts to this book:
the wonderful photographers Billy and Jenny Cardoni, Dimitri Halkidis,
David Webber, Bud Struck, Waring Abbott, Pauline St. Denis, Meghan Boody;
designer Ronni Ascagni for her skilled art direction and Patricia Stein
for her help and assistance; Susan Blinkhorn and Tara Milutis for their research;
Melanie Menagh for her writing and knowledge; makeup artists Jo-Ann DiLorenzo
and Nancy Sprague; stylist Barbra Jerard; and Primavera Boma-Brehram
and Dennis Solay for their beautiful accessories.

To models Francine Tint,
Claudine Thomas, Baret Boisson, Mila Radulovic,
and the women from around the world whose images
grace these pages: you are all great beauties.

A million thanks to naturopath Barbara Close,
trichologist Phillip Kingsley, and yoga instructor Dr. Joe Caraccilo
for their invaluable help and information.

Thanks go to lawyers Richard Hofstetter and Brad Hoylman,
for their hard work and advice, and to Jill Goodacre Connick, Kathy Ireland, and Group 3.

Very special thanks and deepest gratitude to Alex Tart and Charles Miers
at Universe Publishing for believing and sharing in my vision to create a book
of beauty and holistic health from around the world.

And, finally, thanks to Ted Duff for all your understanding and patience.

To all the native american people,
Every creature and part of the Earth was sacred.
It was their belief that to waste or destroy nature
and its wonders was to destroy Life itself.
Their words were not understood in their time.
Now they haunt us. Before it is too late we must listen.

Susan Jefferies
from "Brother Eagle, Sister Sky" 1992

For indigenous peoples, Life and Earth are synonymous.
The Earth is our foundation, the source of our spirituality,
the foundation from which our cultures and language flourish.
The Earth is the keeper of events and the bones of our forefathers,
the substantial evidence of our people's existence before memory.
The Earth is our historian, our educator, the provider of food, medicine,
clothing, and protection. She is the Mother of our races.
Nature is a legacy we leave our children.

Marcus Colchester
an Indian from a tribe in the rainforest

Never doubt that a small group of thoughtfully committed citizens can change the world. Indeed it is the only thing that ever has.

Margaret Mead